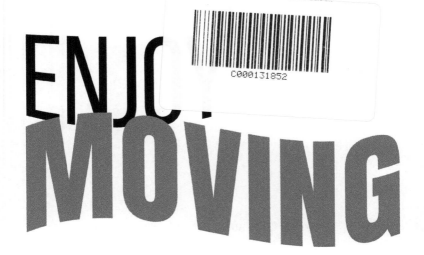

ENJOY
MOVING

AND
FEEL
FABULOUS!

**A Pilates
Lifestyle for
Busy Women**

GILA ARCHER

Cover image by: Rita Sriharningsih
Book design by: SWATT Books Ltd

Printed in the United Kingdom
First Printing, 2022

ISBN: 978-1-7390983-0-8 (Paperback)
ISBN: 978-1-7390983-1-5 (eBook)

Jigsaw Publishing
Chesterfield, Derbyshire, S45 9PH

www.gilaarcherpilates.com

Praise for 'Enjoy Moving & Feel Fabulous'

"I have always struggled with exercise in my life, which stems from being picked last in PE lessons, it set my belief that exercise was something I was not good at and should avoid. I think that's why I relate to Gila's approach and why it's easy to get on board with. Movement is the key message, leaving exercise out of it. Gila shows you how easy it is to engage with short sessions of Pilates and get movement back into your life The result is that I now seek out space in the day to get onto the mat."

Tracie Tipper, Business woman, Mum and CORE Member

"What a breath of fresh air!

This book has really helped me reframe my feelings about and experiences of exercise, moving from those awful memories of school P.E. lessons to helping me recognise how important movement is in my life.

It also made me see how I use being 'busy' as a valid reason why I don't do things for myself.

This is not simply a book about Pilates, this is an essential read for any woman who knows she's not putting herself first."

Joanne Manville, Entrepreneur, Mum and CORE Member

"Gila has huge insight into why ordinary busy women struggle to fit exercise and movement into their lives. Following her pragmatic steps, I was very quickly able to see what obstacles were in my way and, crucially, how to overcome them. With the book still by my side, Gila continues to mentor me through my journey in becoming the best version of myself!"

Lara Ross, Entrepreneur, Mum and CORE Member

"As a successful womanpreneur with over 20 years running multiple 6 and 7 figure businesses and juggling being a mummy to four children, I know how difficult it can be for busy women to prioritise their own self care, health and fitness. We all know how important it is for our mental and physical health to exercise yet it is often not a priority simply due to time and that long to do list that never seems to end.

I met Gila several years ago on a business retreat I was leading and saw first-hand her passion for and knowledge of movement and Pilates. It has been a pleasure to see her turn her expertise into a unique approach that helps busy women make moving and exercising easy and enjoyable.

Her awesome book is a must read for any busy woman who is trying to juggle work and family life always feeling they have no time for themselves. Gila takes you through practical steps and strategies, giving you the tools to implement Pilates into your lifestyle. Not only does she encourage you to get up and moving – as you'd expect – but she also challenges your thinking, sharing her own stories and those of women she has helped.

By taking that first step and reading this book, you will begin your journey from busy woman with no time to exercise, to a woman who loves moving, a woman who is committed to looking after herself as much as looking after everyone else."

Jo Davison, Founder of the Womanpreneur Success Club.

"Fascinating, heart-warming, incredibly informative and a joy to read are just a few words to describe this incredible book. I have loved reading every last bit. This book has been written by a real person from the heart with real, everyday women juggling life, family and career in mind.

It is full of true, inspiring stories and wonderful transformations that are a pleasure to read. Practical advice based on scientific information she has given is so fascinating. I have learned so much about my body and how it evolved from early years to old age in this book. I learned a thing or two about true self-care. Most importantly of all, I have learned how to look after my body by simple, tangible and very practical exercises Gila provides in her book. It is a must-read for a busy woman who lost their true identity in being someone for everyone else. If you are one of these women, then give yourself the gift to read this book and learn to enjoy moving and feel fabulous again, because by the end of this book you will!"

Dr. Tülay Massey, Mindset Transformation Coach

Table of Contents

Disclaimer

You should consult with a general practitioner before beginning any exercises or fitness regime especially if you are pregnant, given birth within the last 6 weeks or have a pre-existing health condition. Your performance of any exercises or movements described in the book are solely at your own risk.

I am not a medical practitioner nor a scientist. Move mindfully, listening to your body. Nothing should be painful. If it is, seek the advice of your doctor.

If you experience any sore muscles, often a day or two after exercising, then this is generally a good sign that you have worked your muscles and are building strength.

All names have been changed to respect people's privacy.

The recommendations in this book are based on my own experience and that of working with other women.

Foreword

*G*ila is a fellow business owner who I met in a business coaching group about 20 months ago. We connected straightaway whilst in this group and helped support each other in our business endeavours. Our relationship grew stronger over these months through supporting each other in various activities online. I first properly encountered Gila's teaching when I gave a talk about the power of our words in her membership group.

About 6 months ago, Gila enrolled in my coaching programme. This is when I really got to know the real Gila. I was with her during her journey of writing this book and when I had the chance to read it before launch I was thrilled.

Nothing had prepared me for the thoughts and feelings this book has created in me whilst reading it. From the moment I started reading it, it was as if she was talking to me. I could picture myself in every situation she described and every struggle she went through. Even though we had different lives, grew up in different places, countries in my case, I could totally relate to everything she is talking about. Everything she wrote about is her real and true experience; and every single woman who has to juggle life, family, a job or a business can relate to what she is saying.

Gila helped me look at myself and how I see self-care in a whole new light, even in the first few pages of this book. The advice you will read is different to anything you will see elsewhere. She makes it so simple, tangible and doable, because she knows how hard it is for a busy woman like her, like me and like you to give our power and energy away to everyone and everything else we 'have to do' until there is no life left in us. Looking after yourself doesn't even come into it and when it does, it normally involves crashing down in front of the TV with a glass (or two) of something.

It often may even involve 'doing nothing' to deal with aches and pains triggered by various daily activities you and I are doing wrong without being aware of it (e.g. sitting for a long time in the same position, not moving our body in the right way, or not moving at all)!

In her book Gila breaks down all the norms of cramming hard-core exercise into your daily life. Instead, she gives the reader easy, doable, bitesize implementable steps you can take at any time of day no matter what your lifestyle is. In this book, Gila helped me understand the root cause of some of this pain and how to get rid of it through gentle and regular exercise that is in tune with my body. I know so many people who still believe they cannot exercise or move their body until they are free of pain, without realising the pain is caused mainly by not moving their body in the first place. If you are one of these people, this book will change your life!

Gila is the perfect person to write such a book, because she has a lifetime of experience in moving her body as a professional gymnast (since the age of 3). She also trained as a professional physical education teacher and a physical development coach, helping people from all ages in developing their body and their confidence through physical exercise. She is a level 4 Pilates instructor, which is the highest qualification to be had in this field. But most importantly of all, she has lived ever single moment of her life going through and overcoming the struggles she has written in her book.

This book is particularly relevant to busy women who juggle family life, career and/or business, who have lost their identity to being everything for everyone else and have lost themselves in their to-do list. We often don't appreciate what we have until we lose it. Losing your ability to move, just because you don't know how, could be devastating not just for you but for those who depend on you. Give yourself the gift of moving your body and truly enjoying the miracle that you live in by being a healthy, happy and active version of yourself!

It will truly change your life and the life of those who depend on you! Happy reading!

Dr. Tülay Massey, Mindset Transformation Coach

Introduction

*H*i, I'm Gila (pronounced with a 'g' as in 'gorilla' – gee-la). I'll tell you that now, because people always ask me.

The other question I always get asked is: "That's an unusual name – where is it from?"

Well, I've been told lots of different things over the years, and although there is actually a lizard called a 'Gila Monster' that has a poisonous bite, I prefer to stick with the story my parents told me, that they heard the name, believed it originated from Japan and means 'The Trusted One'.

I'm not going to tell you my life story – you'll hear snippets through this book anyway, but I will tell you three things about myself that may surprise you.

1. I am not a fitness fanatic! I do not live and breathe exercise every minute of the day. Any exercise or activity I do is because I enjoy doing it and it enables me to do lots of other things I enjoy too. I exercise so I can live, not live to exercise.

2. I am a 'normal' woman, the same as you. I'm not perfect. I make mistakes, get things wrong, wobble when trying to balance, have good days and not-so-good days. I am about feeling good in myself. I don't do exercise to get a 6-pack or a big bootie! However, I know that if I enjoy moving and feel fabulous about myself, I will also look fabulous! I want to look great, of course I do, but you won't find me posting a selfie of me in my bikini on social media! I am about feeling healthy, confident and calm, and being the best version of me I can be. The rest will fall into place.

3. I don't drink alcohol or tea or coffee – not for any health reasons – but because I just don't like them. My weakness is chocolate! Any chocolate really, except really cheap stuff! I probably eat it most days! Once a box is open – I just can't help myself!!! As a client once said to me, when I asked her what was good about my Pilates class, she replied, "It's a whole hour when I can't eat any chocolate!" Well, the same goes for me too!

I have always loved moving my body and seeing what I was capable of physically and mentally, but when I struggled for several years to keep movement and exercise in my life, I felt unhappy and discontented in myself. This led me to discover a different approach to movement, one that I could easily and enjoyably fit into my lifestyle, with 3 children, a dog and several businesses to run.

In this book I am excited to share with you my philosophy and approach to movement, that enables me to remain strong, flexible, feel good about myself AND still enjoy everything else that is important to me. Joseph Pilates had a very similar philosophy about movement and the health of the human body and Pilates is an essential tool in my approach.

It's not magic!

WARNING

You will not suddenly become superwoman, gain a 6-pack, be able to do the splits, get your bikini body, look like a supermodel or even sit at your desk without your back aching just by reading this book. It's not magic!

This is not meant to be another book to just look pretty on the bookshelf, for a rainy day or to read and not take action. It is also not just information you can find anywhere else.

This book is about my growth and evolution to develop my unique approach to keeping fit whilst being a busy woman. The same approach that many busy women now use successfully and easily to look after their physical and mental health whilst also juggling families, careers and life in general.

I have intentionally written this book in small, manageable chunks so you can just read a little bit at a time. You can read it in the car whilst waiting to pick the children up from school, or even in the bath, or for 5 minutes each night before bed, it's up to you.

Throughout the book there are **'Get Moving'** and **'Get Thinking'** boxes, where I want you to take action and begin to shift your thinking and move your body.

I'd encourage you to complete each of the tasks and practise the movements as you go along. This book can be your journal, so use it, write in it, draw in it, take it everywhere you go! Take time to reflect on your thoughts, dig deeper and take action before reading the next section. Let this book become your companion to support you in your journey to become your best self.

Imagine it is a bit like having me with you in your pocket! This was in fact something a good friend and client said to me recently – that she'd just "love a mini-Gila to keep in my pocket and bring out whenever I need some motivation and help". Well, this is for her – and you – she knows who she is!

So, you have two choices when reading this book – flick through it and decide you are too busy to take any action and then nothing will change

OR

Prove to yourself you have got the time to read this, think about it and take the necessary action. You can decide to commit 100% and it will then be easy to make the changes you desire and achieve those fitness goals that keep eluding you.

This book will change your life. This may seem like a bold statement to make, but what I am sharing with you in this book changed my life and the lives of so many other busy women I've had the honour and privilege to work with who have followed my approach and taken action. We have all learnt, grown and evolved to live our lives on purpose, with choice and feel fabulous about ourselves. This is what I want for you too.

> *"Physical fitness is not acquired through wishful thinking or outright purchase"*
>
> Joseph Pilates, 1945

Enjoy this book and your journey!

Gila x

Chapter 1

Born to move, not exercise

*I*f you think exercise is time-consuming, unnatural and really just a form of punishment, you may not be far wrong!

The good old days

My nanna (my dad's mum) is 100 years old and counting, and she believes firmly that she grew up in the best era. She lives on her own, is independent, climbs the stairs each night to go to bed, cooks her own meals, continues to peel all the apples from her trees in her garden (that she grew from seeds by the way) to use in apple pies and apple crumbles. She refuses to have a cordless phone (she calls it a mobile), so when the phone rings, she gets up and walks to answer the phone – when she can hear it! As far as I know, she has never done any 'exercise classes' in her life – but has always kept moving.

My dad often recalls how he used to play cricket in the road outside his house. My children find this really strange, because now, when we visit Nanna, you can only get down the road if nothing is coming the other way because cars are parked on each side.

Even I, and I'm not that old, remember walking to school every day. I also remember playing with a long piece of elastic stretched between two concrete bollards at the end of our cul-de-sac, jumping over the elastic, feet jumping in-between, on, right and left of the elastic as we chanted different rhymes.

Do you remember walking to school, playing in the street with your friends, getting up off the sofa to change the TV channel, standing by the phone to take a call, drawing a chalk hopscotch on the pavement and walking to the shops and carrying your shopping home? None of this was 'exercise'. This was movement! It was part of our natural life. This is part of how we used to keep healthy.

Exercise, as a voluntary form of movement that we undertake for health and fitness benefits, is a modern invention, because the movement opportunities available in our habitual lifestyles have got less and less, not just in the last 100 years, but dramatically so since the time when we evolved as a human species, and evolutionarily speaking our bodies have not adapted adequately. Lieberman (2021)

Whether or not you agree that the good old days were the best ones to grow up in, it would benefit us all to acknowledge and be aware that as our way of living changes, there will be advantages and disadvantages.

As you will of course know, there are numerous health benefits for remaining physically active.

'Physical inactivity is one of the leading risk factors for noncommunicable diseases (NCDs) and death worldwide. It increases the risk of cancer, heart disease, stroke and diabetes by 20-30%. It is estimated that four to five million deaths per year could be averted if the global population was more active. One in four adults – and four out of five adolescents don't do enough physical activity. Women and girls generally are less active than men and boys, widening health inequalities.'
World Health Organisation

However, there are more benefits to moving than just our physical health. Our movement has an impact on how we develop physically, mentally, socially and cognitively from the moment we are born.

I remember someone saying to me once as a passing comment, "Oh, you've got lovely handwriting, that's because you are a gymnast. Gymnasts always have neat handwriting."

I can't remember who said it, but what they said intrigued me to find out if there was any truth in it. Do gymnasts always have neat handwriting and if so, why?

This question is what started my interest and passion in the importance of movement.

I researched the impact of a gymnastic-based movement programme on the cognitive development (including handwriting) of a child with poor motor co-ordination. I ran an 'Esteem Club', so called because the focus was on developing and improving children's physical co-ordination and self-esteem. I worked with many children and their parents in my school and across the county and spoke about my work at headteachers' conferences and at the International Physical Literacy Conference.

The boy with Velcro shoes

John joined Esteem Club when he was about 12 years old. He was my height, had poor muscle tone, was quiet and nervous. I could tell upon meeting him that he struggled to keep control of his body. The way he walked was laboured, his running was slow and heavy. He wasn't able to hop on one leg – this is in fact a complex skill which requires strength, balance and co-ordination but should be able to be performed by the time a child is 3-5 years old. Gallahue and Ozmun (1995) He spoke slowly and you had to listen carefully to what he said as it wasn't very clear. You see, even speaking requires the co-ordination of your tongue in your mouth to make the right sounds. (Dyspraxia Foundation)

John's mum had explained that he got upset at school because he was teased for having Velcro shoes. He couldn't tie his shoelaces. It may not be obvious until you stop to think about it but tying shoelaces requires core stability to hold the body still, whatever position you are in, so that then your arms can remain steady, and you have control over the fine motor movements required of your hands and fingers. You also need well-developed spatial awareness to understand the shapes the laces make and how they move around each other.

John loved coming to Esteem Club because he felt like he wasn't the only one. He felt like he belonged, and he made friends, something he hadn't really done before. He didn't go to any other clubs and would often remove himself from social situations in the playground to avoid being teased or making a fool of himself.

He was a very kind boy with amazingly supportive parents, who practised the movements with him at home too. During one conversation with his mum, she shared with me that he had never crawled as a baby; he had just sat up and then walked. Now, as a parent, it would be very easy to focus on this achievement of walking and it is certainly a milestone worth celebrating. However, through my research and that of others, notably Sally Goddard Blythe MSc., author, lecturer and International Director of The Institute for Neuro-Physiological Psychology, the crawling stage of a child's physical development is a crucial step. Crawling builds pelvic and shoulder stability, core strength, cross patterning, co-ordination and helps to release the palmar grasp reflex, which is an involuntary movement that is seen in babies up to about 6 months. (This is the reflex when you place your finger into a baby's palm and they close their fingers around yours and grip on tightly.) Crawling also strengthens the arms and thighs and trains the eyes at the optimum distance for reading and writing. Nearly all children I have worked with over the years who had a marked delay in their motor co-ordination had missed out on the crawling stage of their physical development.

So, I can still remember clearly, when John was 15 years old, he stood up in front of the group, spoke clearly and confidently and told us how he had achieved his first belt at karate club. I still feel emotional now, thinking about it. I had a lump in my throat, I was so proud of him. By this stage, he could tie his shoelaces, do up buttons and his school tie, no problem. The transformation in him was huge and I feel very privileged to have been able to help him at this stage in his life. Improving his physical development, core strength and gross motor skills had a ripple effect on his fine motor skills, his speech and his confidence.

What has crawling got to do with handwriting?

Olivia was kind and gentle but was always banging into everything and everyone in the classroom when she moved around. She was tall for her age, wore thick glasses and some people might have seen her and then described her as 'clumsy'. She lacked spatial and body awareness, and this would annoy other children when she unintentionally invaded their space. When sitting next to someone she would spread right across the table, almost laying across it, because she lacked the core strength and endurance to sit up in her chair. This would inevitably result in pens and books being pushed across the desk and onto the floor. She was always the last one changed for PE because she struggled with buttons, zips and getting dressed.

As a result of poor core strength, Olivia was not able to sit up automatically and so struggled to control her shoulder stability and therefore had poor control over her fine motor skills and her handwriting. She was 9 years old when she was in my class, and her handwriting was huge and illegible. She had been diagnosed with Developmental Co-ordination Disorder and had missed important physical milestones, one of them crawling.

Now, the answer to improving her handwriting was NOT to do MORE handwriting. The problem was not her lack of fine motor control, it went deeper than that. She needed to gain control of her gross motor skills and core body strength first, then she would be able to better control her arm and hand to write. (Goddard Blythe (2009), Gallahue and Ozmun (1995), Dyspraxia Foundation)

Instead, I invited her to Esteem Club and got her crawling and pushing up from the floor on her front, flattening her hand out on the floor, strengthening her core and shoulder stability. She practised balancing on one leg and walking in a straight line and many other exercises specific to improving her core strength, stability, and body and spatial awareness. Again, her parents were very supportive and did exercises with her at home too. (If you've done Pilates before, you'd definitely recognise the exercises and movements I was doing with these children. Joseph Pilates understood the importance of core strength).

By the time Olivia was 10 years old her handwriting had improved massively, and it was now neat and legible. She moved around the classroom with more care and was getting on better with the children in the class. She was much happier and more confident as a result.

Crawling: the latest fitness craze

The point I want to make is how important movement is, from the minute we are born, to all areas of our life. Not just for our physical development but, as you can see from the examples above, for our cognitive development, social skills and self-esteem too. These are, it goes without saying, important for our health and wellbeing too.

The worrying thing is that, in my time as a teacher and consultant, the number of children I saw who struggled with their gross motor skills, co-ordination and balance, increased.

I would argue that children don't play physically as much as they did a few decades ago. A lot of their play takes place more and more in a virtual world on a screen. I've even seen this in my children, and my husband and I are highly aware of limiting screen time. In the natural kingdom, we see examples of young animals playing physically and naturally, developing their stability, co-ordination and agility. As humans, even though we don't need to hunt for our food anymore, our physical development – stability, co-ordination and agility – remains as essential to our survival as it ever did. I would argue more so. We need to be physically active for our physical and mental health, regardless of the environment we are living in.

The good thing is, it doesn't have to be this way. For the majority of children, who do not have additional needs, just by allowing them more movement opportunities, putting them in different positions as a baby, allowing them to struggle to lift their head off the floor when laying on their front, encouraging them to crawl

– whatever their age, to roll off the sofa, to jump on the bed, to wriggle, squirm, stretch, walk along the wall, roll down a hill, hop over the cracks in the pavement, skip, even lay on their front to read a book, all this will give them the foundation to become physically literate and active throughout their lives. This is supported by other professionals in education and health, Sally Goddard Blythe and Elizabeth Hayden being just two examples.

Even for adults, crawling is a great core strength exercise and builds strength needed for real life. If you search on YouTube, you will actually find crawling workouts you can follow!

Get Moving

Get crawling! Crawl along the floor. How does it feel? How fast can you crawl?

Have a crawling race with your children!

Do you exercise like a hamster?

> *"Did you ever hear of an animal gymnasium*
> *conducted by animals for animals, for*
> *the purpose of gratifying their desire*
> *or need for artificial exercising?"*
>
> Pilates (1934, p30)

Have you ever seen a cat jump on a rowing machine or a dog lifting weights? The closest exercise you may see in animals is a hamster or gerbil running around in a wheel or ball – but that's only because it is no longer in its natural habitat.

A bit like our modern-day lifestyle. We are no longer living in the habitat we evolved in. Our environment is comfortable, we spend much of our time sitting and being inactive and then have to compensate for our lack of movement by doing artificial exercise e.g., running on a treadmill or pedalling on a bike indoors, putting in a lot of effort to go nowhere. Treadmills have been used in history – most notably by the Victorians as a form of punishment for prisoners – not a positive association!

Joseph Pilates spent a lot of time observing how animals moved in the natural world and often made comparisons with cats and how they move and stretch, how they conserve energy, how they hunt and how they maintain perfect (normal) health without exercising.

> *"... one observes the perfection of physical*
> *form, strength, grace, agility, endurance,*
> *health and longevity in the animal kingdom.*
> *With man it is just to the contrary."*
>
> Pilates (1934, p30)

Move to survive

Our ancestors understood this. They had to move to keep warm, find food, escape danger and survive. Movement was an integral part of everything they did – foraging for berries, collecting wood, hunting, making shelters, escaping dangers, bending, walking, running, crouching, squatting, twisting, turning, carrying heavy weights. This is still the case with modern hunter-gatherer tribes that exist in different parts of the world. (Lieberman, 2021)

They do not need to 'exercise', as every movement they make enables them to function efficiently and effectively in order to continue doing everything they need to. We are designed to move, and our body only works properly if we are moving.

Our Western culture is very different. We sit, on average in the UK and USA, for 9.5-10 hours a day. This means many of us could be suffering from The Sitting Disease, 'a term coined by the scientific community and is commonly used when referring to the ill-effects of an overly sedentary lifestyle.' (www.juststand.org)

Sitting, for the spine, is like sugar for the teeth. Sitting for more than 4 hours a day and more than 30 minutes at a time (that includes sitting in a car, to eat, watch TV, work at a computer), is harmful for your health according to countless research and organisations: Just Stand Organisation, Harvard Health, Yale Medicine, The British Heart Foundation, NHS and British Medical Journal.

There are also related signs to watch out for: reduced energy, increased weight gain, poor sleep, poor concentration and memory, reduced productivity, lower mood levels and poor posture, musculoskeletal problems, backache and neck ache. (NHS.UK, Just Stand Organisation, World Health Organisation) If we stay still for too long our whole system breaks down, the damage creeping up on us slowly.

Ants in your pants?

The most pointless thing, in my opinion, to say to a young child is "Sit still". Wriggling around on their bottom, shifting their weight on their seat, changing position all helps them practise balancing and improve their stability. Sitting still and standing still are actually very difficult skills to master.

As a child you are still developing control over your body. The only way to maintain your balance is by moving, as it's virtually impossible to sit completely still. Try it!

Get Moving

If you stand on one leg and close your eyes, you'll feel your supporting leg wobbling, moving side to side, forwards and backwards. This wobbling is good. It is stopping you falling flat on your face, it is your proprioception working, supplying your brain and muscles with constant feedback to keep you upright.

Also, when children fidget (moving their hands and feet or body in small movements, that seemingly have no purpose and they don't realise they are doing it), it helps to keep their blood circulating and carrying oxygen to their brain, which in turn helps them to concentrate and remain focused.

However, it's not that our ancestors never sat. Of course they did. They sat to rest, conserve energy, do some daily tasks and socialise. Importantly, when they sat, they squatted down. (Lieberman, 2021) If you look at young children when they play, they will often do the same. There is no compression on the spine when you squat. Squatting saves a lot of wear and tear on the weaker muscles of the back, and you don't have to lean forward, as the centre of gravity is over the ankles. Squatting is also better when going to the toilet as it allows for easier bowel movements. (www.squattypotty.co.uk)

It is not sitting per se that is the issue. In my opinion it is how we sit and for how long we sit that causes health issues.

Are you sitting comfortably?

Well, don't! Get up and move!

In the UK, and other Western countries, we predominantly sit on chairs. Now, you may wonder what else we would sit on. The problem being that chairs with backs, cushions and support mean we don't have to use our own muscles to hold our bodies.

I always cringe when I see adverts for these jacket type contraptions that you see a model wearing, demonstrating how without it their upper back hunches forwards and they have poor posture but as soon as they put it on over their back and shoulders, they can miraculously stand up tall and straight. 'Never have bad posture again!' Well, in my opinion, they are just selling you your desire for a quick fix.

The long-term solution to standing up straight with good posture is about addressing the root causes of your posture, and one of the causes will be the lack of strength in your back and core. So, the solution to having a good posture is to USE YOUR OWN MUSCLES!

Get Thinking

How long have you sat down today? Count it up, every trip in the car, every minute at your desk, sitting at mealtimes to eat, in the bath, in front of the TV. (www.juststand.org/the-tools/sitting-time-calculator)

As humans, our brains want an easy, comfortable, least amount of effort and immediate solution.

When I was a teacher, I did suggest that children would be better sat on stability balls than chairs, because they would improve their core and back strength, be able to fidget and hence concentrate better. However, it was a leap of faith too far for the schools I worked in at the time. Yet, I'm pleased to see in Bjerkreim School in Rogaland, Norway they have replaced chairs with large stability balls. This hasn't negatively impacted on children's studies, the balls are softer to sit on, cheaper than chairs and the children are benefitting physically and mentally.

(www.thelocal.no/20160321/norway-school-swaps-chairs-for-giant-rubber-balls)

Different cultures sit in different ways. Japan has a tradition of sitting on the floor for tea ceremonies and in India sitting cross-legged or in a lotus position has high spiritual value. Different types of 'chairs' have also been designed, for example, ones that you can kneel on and support your own spine, and even standing desks are now becoming more popular for people working from home and in offices in Western countries, to alternate between sitting and standing.

If your lifestyle involves a lot of sitting, think about how long you are sitting for, what position you are sat in, what you are sat on, and keep moving and taking breaks.

Get Moving

Fidget, wriggle, move, change position, stand up, sit on the floor, cross your legs, squat.

How long can you squat for?

Swap your chair at your desk for one with no back support or try sitting on a stability ball to work.

Stick with it and feel the benefits.

Born with the right to move

The tradition in many countries has always been to 'wear' your baby. Mozambiquan mothers traditionally carry their infants in a piece of printed cotton material called a capulana. Mothers in Africa wrap kangas around their bodies like a towel to carry their babies on their backs. Throughout Mexico, craftswomen wear babies in a rebozo, a long, narrow rectangle of fabric they use to attach their kids to their hips or front of the body.

Women of Colombia strap their new-born to their backs in a large cloth sling with an additional strap that goes around the mother's forehead. In colder climates babies have the advantage of keeping warm wrapped in the mother's own clothing, made of animal fur and sinew. In Nepal, infants have been carried in wicker baskets strapped to the mother's head.

The advantage with 'wearing' your baby is it means you have both hands free to hold other children's hands or carry food/fuel and do other tasks, and the baby has the security of being close to their mother. In respect to movement, all the methods of carrying described above are not rigid, as they allow space for babies to wriggle, move their legs, lift their head, look around and be jostled and rocked around by the movement of their mother. Healthline.com also state it helps with connection, breastfeeding, reduces crying, promotes health and eases everyday life.

In contrast, in Western culture, although slings and wearing our babies has become more popular, we have a different lifestyle. There are laws that babies must be strapped into a car seat, so they are safe when being transported in a car. We can also conveniently transfer the car seat to a buggy, or as I've seen many women do, just carry the car seat at your side as you nip out on a school run or into the post office, back in the car and click onto the Isofix. When you get home, you can carry the car seat inside with baby safely strapped in.

However, all this time, the baby has not had an opportunity to move or change position or wriggle around. They have remained in a semi-flexed position; their body supported. And as for the mother, whilst still regaining her core strength and recovering from pregnancy and giving birth, she may be trying to carry a car seat at her side. Have you ever tried this? It is not only awkward but requires a lot of shoulder strength to stop it banging into your leg, your posture is unsymmetrical, and you're not only carrying the weight of the baby but the weight of the car seat as well.

Babies are strapped in car seats, highchairs and buggies for safety but can remain in these positions for longer periods of time than necessary to suit our convenience. This restricts their natural movement development.

Even the World Health Organisation has recognised the lack of movement opportunities our young children have, stating:

'Children under five must spend less time sitting watching screens, or restrained in prams and seats, get better quality sleep and have more time for active play if they are to grow up healthy.'

By 'wearing' your baby in a sling or similar it is not only better for their physical development but means a mother can look after herself better too. I have a number of clients who have sought my help to rebalance poor posture and backache from having to lift heavy car seats out of a car, or from carrying babies repeatedly in a car seat.

Tummy Time

After having each of my children, I was advised by the midwife not to lay my baby on their front to sleep because of dangers related to cot death. The American Academy of Paediatrics recommended the 'Back to Sleep' Campaign to reduce the incident of Sudden Infant Death Syndrome in 1994. It has been extremely successful and has decreased the rates of SIDS by almost 50%. (safetosleep.nichd.nih.gov/activities/campaign)

I know from my own work that this message was so powerful it resulted in scaring many mothers into placing their babies on their tummies even when awake and if they did, as soon as they cried, they'd pick them up. In addition, paediatricians began to see an increase in skull deformities that they attributed to the increase in infants laying on their backs. (Persing et al (2003) and Argenta et al (1996)) Osteopath Elizabeth Hayden, in her book *Osteopathy for Children* also advocates prone laying and movement to aid in the development of the spine.

'Tummy Time' was created in response to the 'Back to Sleep' campaign to advocate and promote front laying for babies when they are awake and supervised. In support of this, research has shown that babies who spend more time awake on their tummies reach gross motor skill milestones, for example rolling over and crawling, earlier than babies who were regularly placed on their backs to sleep. However, although this delay is observed in other research, it is not significant enough to change the now 'Safe to Sleep' message. (Dewey et al (1998), Godard-Blythe (2008), NCT.org.uk)

"What's most important is that kids be in a variety of positions during the day," said Dr Jill Heathcock, Ph.D., a researcher who studies early motor development at Ohio State University, (www.nytimes.com/2020/04/13/parenting/baby/tummy-time) and I agree. At the end of my teaching day, when I read a story on the carpet, I would allow any children who wanted to lay on their front, propped on their elbows, to listen to the story. I found they were able to listen better and without their knowing they were building their shoulder stability at the same time!

Just think about the impact a comfortable and convenient lifestyle is having on the movement opportunities, development and physical health of ourselves and the next generation.

If it's easy, then it's probably not Pilates!

I recognise that I was brought up in an active family and given so many opportunities to do different activities in and outside school.

Your experiences of being active at school and home will have given you beliefs about yourself and your relationship with exercise, which is likely to influence your attitude towards moving. You may well have a different cultural background to me, will have had a different upbringing and of course will have had different life experiences, different role models, which all add up to form your mindset about exercise.

Your experience of games lessons at school may be similar to mine. I was on the hockey squad at secondary school – goodness knows why. I was tiny, shy and quiet. I played in defence. One advantage was that because I was on the squad the ball hardly ever came up my end of the pitch. The problem with that, though, was I just got cold and miserable. I really didn't enjoy my games lessons as a result. But you may have loved this opportunity and have been playing up at the front.

Get Thinking

What was your experience of PE, sport and physical activity as you were growing up? What are your beliefs about being active now and do you think your beliefs now stem from your experiences earlier on in your life?

You may enjoy sport, playing squash or netball, but don't like to exercise.

'Exercise' is adapted from the Latin verb 'exerceo' meaning 'keep busy' which is ironic because we find ourselves today often without time to exercise because we are too busy. Doing exercise takes up time and can feel like a chore. Is that because it's not natural for humans to exercise or because of what we've been conditioned to believe?

For example, I have a few clients who tell themselves they are going to 'move' today because that in their mind has a more pleasurable and easier association than the word 'exercise'. I know other women who love playing sport and team games and would call themselves 'sporty' but still see 'exercise' as something they 'should' do rather than something they 'want' to do.

I even have a sweatshirt that says, 'If it's easy, then it's probably not Pilates!' and at a surface level we can laugh at this, and you'll often see implications in quotes etc that Pilates is hard.

I get this to a point. When you do Pilates correctly, you will gain so much. You will:

- strengthen and lengthen your muscles effectively
- move your body through the barrier of tightness and stiffness
- need to concentrate on what you are doing to get the most from it
- be sore in a way that you know your muscles are getting stronger

However, if we keep telling ourselves something will be hard, then it will be. If you believe it will be easy, then it will be.

On the flipside, some women like to feel like they've 'worked hard', 'worked out' when they exercise and enjoy pushing themselves. Me too, to a point. I like to challenge my body and mind to see what I'm actually capable of. I don't go in for ultramarathons, running across the desert or have any desire to break the world record for a woman of holding the plank (which is over 4 hours by the way), but I do love a challenge.

At the end of the day, whether it is sport or exercise or physical activity it is all movement. Moving is good for the body and the mind.

Whatever it is, find something you enjoy doing. Whatever we call it, whatever our upbringing, whatever our cultural background, whatever our natural strengths and weaknesses, we were all born to move.

In many respects, there are more movement opportunities for girls today. The range of sports, exercise and physical activity open to girls and women today has increased. More girls are playing football or taking up boxing thanks to role models like Nicola Adams. Surfing, skateboarding and climbing are now included in the Olympics for women.

I advocate moving in a way you enjoy. Then you want to do it, it is no longer a chore or something you feel you should do. It's not a punishment, it feels good and natural, and so you'll be happier investing your time in moving. I don't see Pilates as 'exercise'. I don't do it because I tell myself I should. *I do Pilates, ballet, aerial silks and walking because I want to, because I enjoy it.*

I enjoy moving my body.

Get Thinking

1. Which words have a positive association for you? (Physical activity, exercise, fitness, sport, workout, movement)

2. What movement do you ENJOY doing?

Just keep moving until you reach 100

So why does movement matter for us as busy women?

Well, for all the same reasons as to why it matters for a child to move. Humans evolved to move, to be active, not to exercise. Because our habitat has now changed and we are not naturally as active, we need to find a new way of moving that enables us to still thrive and survive in our modern environment.

> *'We evolved to be physically active as we age, and in turn being active helps us age well. Further, the longer we stay active, the greater the benefit, and it is almost never too late to benefit from getting fit.'*
>
> Lieberman (2021, p251)

Lieberman describes many observations and studies he has conducted on hunter-gatherer communities, one being the Hadza community in North Tanzania, and reports how the men and women both remain physically active as they get older, which benefits the whole community.

> *"Thanks to an active lifestyle without retirement, there is no significant age-related decline in walking speed among Hadza women, whose average pace remains a brisk 3.6 feet per second well into their seventies."*
>
> Lieberman (2021, p233)

The fact is we are all getting older all the time, and this is out of our control. But if we stop moving, we age quicker. Our muscle mass decreases, we become weaker, our vision decreases, our balance decreases, we are more prone to falls and injuries, our bodies gradually deteriorate. Physical activity is not the Holy Grail but helps us age well. If we want to, at the very least, maintain our health and movement capabilities, the incidental movement we get from our sedentary, modern, comfortable living is not enough.

Since forever, people have tried ways to stay younger and live longer and the most sensible advice has always mentioned movement. We all know, and numerous research confirms this, that regular physical activity helps extend life. Hippocrates (460-375 BCE) recognised the importance of physical activity on our health:

> ## *"Eating alone will not keep a man well, he must also take exercise."*
> Hippocrates

To maintain our health today, we need to do movements that help rebalance the poor postures and habits we are prone to in this modern living, such as text neck or forward head posture, round shoulders and repetitive strain injuries in our wrist and shoulders.

We need to do movement that specifically strengthens our glutes (bottom) and hip flexors, that gives our spine space and freedom to move after the compression from sitting all day. We need to improve blood circulation after periods of inactivity, so our breathing and blood supply doesn't stagnate. We need to stretch the front and back of our thighs, that have been stuck in one position, strengthen our core so we can move easily without our back hurting, strengthen our upper back and open our chests so we can breathe properly after sitting hunched forward over a desk, and close our eyes and focus on our breath, so our eyes and our mind can rest from staring at screens all day and then focus on ourselves.

The answer?

Pilates

Joseph Pilates was ahead of his time when he designed his 'exercise system' with modern life in mind. This was in the 1940s and since then our lifestyle has only become even more lacking in movement. I'm sure Pilates would have something to say about our inactive lifestyles today – I don't think he would recognise it as 'normal life'.

> *"That in the cause of our daily activities, if we live a normal life, we receive the benefit of natural exercises – those performed in every movement we make. These very necessary functional activities, experienced by one living a normal life, preclude all necessity for undertaking artificial exercise of any kind.'*
>
> Pilates (1934, p29)

I agree with Joseph Pilates but would argue that in the last 80 years we have lost a huge amount of the everyday functional movement that made artificial exercise unnecessary. 'Artificial exercise' has become and needs to become more so, a part of our 'normal', natural way of life. It is then no longer 'artificial exercise' but 'natural movement' – just a new 'natural'.

We need to move more, move specifically to address the habits of a fast-paced technological society, and that movement needs to be consistent and regular, little and often, so we can survive and thrive as human beings today and for the next generation.

In the Western world you may not be able to escape working from a computer at a desk or driving to work or school, but that doesn't mean you cannot remain physically active and integrate natural, conscious movement into your everyday lifestyle.

Your next steps

A good place to start is by moving more and I'm sure you'll be familiar with tips such as taking the stairs instead of the lift, parking further away and walking, and alternating sitting and standing when working from a desk.

But as much as this will help, it is not enough to counteract the amount of inactivity we now have in our lifestyles.

Therefore, it is so important to find a physical activity you enjoy and actually want to do, because you are then more likely to actually do it. For me it's Pilates and it may be for you too.

I'd recommend Pilates for several reasons.

1. Pilates is more than just a man's name. Joseph Pilates called his approach to movement and exercise 'Contrology'. The principles of Pilates that he developed are a way of living.

Pilates is not just something you do whilst in a class for an hour. The principles of movement you learn, your understanding of your body, how to move, how to hold yourself, how to recruit the right muscles etc can be applied to every move you make, whether sitting, gardening, decorating, shopping, carrying children, driving, putting shoes on, lifting, walking, running.

2. Pilates movements require you to move your body in different ways, through different planes of movement, working small muscle groups as well as larger ones. It works muscles you never knew you had!

3. Pilates is about improving the quality of your movement, not the quantity. It is far better to do fewer repetitions of a movement but do these to the best of your ability, thinking about how you are moving your body, encouraging your range of movement to increase, and challenging your body and mind to achieve better. Less is more when it comes to Pilates, which means it is the perfect movement for busy women because it can easily fit into a hectic schedule.

You can of course do more and different activities or sports that you enjoy, but Pilates will give you a solid foundation and core strength whether you take part in other activities or not.

It can become part of your natural way of moving and living and enable you to live a more active life even as you get older. Your age is then irrelevant.

And for busy women there are some benefits of moving and doing Pilates specifically that are extremely good for us. So, Pilates:

- ~ Allows you to do short bitesize workouts which are just as effective as doing an hour of high intensity exercise
- ~ Helps to prevent injuries
- ~ Increases circulation and oxygen-rich blood to the brain which helps overcome fatigue
- ~ Releases endorphins, the feel-good chemicals
- ~ Strengthens pelvic floor muscles, which is important whether we've had children or not, to avoid any embarrassment as we get older
- ~ Helps recovery from diastasis recti (the separation between your rectus abdominal muscles that can happen during pregnancy)
- ~ Gives us the opportunity to focus on ourselves and in doing so let go of all the busyness of the day
- ~ Improves our lung capacity
- ~ Reduces anxiety and improves mood
- ~ Improves posture
- ~ Increases core strength and flattens that mummy tummy
- ~ Strengthens our immune system through an efficient circulation and lymphatic system
- ~ Improves spinal health
- ~ Increases confidence and self-esteem
- ~ Improves flexibility
- ~ Develops greater mobility

So, if there are all these benefits, many of which I'm sure you will already know, why don't we exercise, or exercise more?

The problem is overcoming our natural disinclinations to move and exercise when there are so many other distractions that may not be as good for us but are easy, pleasurable and take up our time.

This is where my approach to movement is designed to help busy women living in the Western world, whose fitness feels like a chore on their never-ending to-do list, to live a physically active and fulfilling life. Through my 'Best Empowered Self Triangle', you have the tools and strategies to enjoy moving and feel fabulous in an easy and achievable way.

Chapter 2

Do you want it enough?

Why I chose Pilates

This was it! Years of practice, 20 years in fact – could I do it? Would I succeed?

I was stood, ready to walk on and present to the judges. Feeling nervous, palms clammy, even though they were covered in chalk, my heart racing, armpits sweating. I was wearing a black, red and yellow velour leotard, matching my two partners, hair was slicked back, solid with hairspray so it didn't dare fall out. We were competing at the National Finals Sports Acrobatics Gymnastics competition, in Stoke on Trent, as a Women's Trio.

The previous trio had just finished their sparklingly perfect routine and were waiting for their score. The thought that went through my head as they walked off was: "They're really tiny. They must only be 8 or 9 years old."

I was 23, which for a gymnast is fairly old. I'd just started working as a primary school teacher and was training every evening.

But my age was irrelevant. The judges did not care. It was how well we performed our routine. We performed it the best we had ever performed it and came 4th. We didn't drop a single balance; we all landed our individual tumbles and the choreography (which I had created) we performed in synchronisation with the music (artistry is also judged).

4th – some may say the worst position, but I disagree. 4th in the country was an achievement to be proud of. We'd already won several previous competitions to even get to this point.

We were already winners, we had already succeeded, we were just taking it to the next level.

However, it was after this competition that I decided to hang up my leotards and coach gymnastics instead. The intense training, a minimum of 8 hours a week, felt like it was getting harder, my body didn't bounce back as quickly as it had 10 years before, and I decided I'd enjoy coaching.

But you know what, my body went from 8 hours of flexibility training, conditioning, repeating skills and balances, sitting in over-splits for minutes on end, doing handstand press-ups until it felt like your wrists would never bend back in the right direction, someone pushing my back down so my chest would touch the floor in straddle, partners climbing up my legs and back to balance on my shoulders leaving bruises on my thighs, to... nothing. Absolutely nothing.

I'd stopped training. I'd stopped moving.

It wasn't until then that I realised how important movement was to me and my body. I had done gymnastics and ballet, tap, modern, jazz etc since I was 3 years old. In my teenage years training more than 14 hours a week.

I was now a primary school teacher during the day and coached gymnastics in the evening and for the first time in my life my back started aching. Not in the way it aches after you've trained hard, that's a good ache, the muscles telling you they are growing stronger, but in a niggly, persistent, dull way.

I knew I had to keep active, but I wanted to find something that I enjoyed without the pressure of competing or performing. That's when I found Pilates.

I started going to an evening class and the teacher said to me, "You are very good at this. Could you teach my class when I'm away?"

"Absolutely! I'd love to", I replied.

I did Pilates classes for me and started teaching odd classes too. I loved it. It gave me the opportunity to still strengthen and condition my body, stretch and mobilise my body, challenge my mind in a different way and switch off from my day job. It has been a part of life ever since – that was in 2001.

Before I share with you my wonderful way of incorporating mindful movement into your life, I'd like you to consider for a moment if you are ready to make a commitment to yourself.

Get Moving

Stand up, bend your knees in as deep a squat as you can and straighten your knees, rise onto your toes, find your balance, hold for a moment and lower your heels.

Repeat 8 times

Did you do it?

Feel better? Just that small amount of movement will increase your circulation and get fresh oxygen-rich blood to your brain and help you continue to concentrate on the next part of this book!

What are you willing to give up?

Are you ready? Are you going to commit 100%, go all-in and give yourself permission to do this for you? Many motivational fitness self-help books and influencers will ask you, 'What are you willing to sacrifice?'

Are you willing to give up watching your favourite TV programme to do Pilates instead?

Are you willing to do your Pilates workout instead of catching a coffee with your friends?

For most of us, we live in a comfortable, technological world, that is fast-paced, and we love convenience. We are always looking for ways to make our life easier and how to avoid anything that is difficult or uncomfortable. We want quick fixes and solutions handed to us on a silver plate. We want to reap our rewards without having to sow the seeds or tend to the crops.

We'd love to be paid thousands of pounds without having to do any work wouldn't we? We'd love to be able to eat what we want without putting on weight, right? Even better, if someone could invent a magic pill that we could just take that made us strong, fit and healthy with no aches or pains without having to do any exercise – would you take it?

Silly question, right?

Have you ever looked at someone else and said: "I'd give anything to be able to... look like them/have their house/be able to run as fast as them/do what they can do?

Have you ever looked at a principal ballerina and said I'd give anything to dance like her or looked at a gymnast and said I'd do anything to be as flexible as her?

Anything?

Would you give up TV, wine, chocolate, crisps, social media?

Or something bigger...

Time?
Energy?
Attention?
Money?
Other people's approval?

Everyone wants to be successful until they see what it takes. And then most change their mind and realise they don't really want to be that successful, they'd rather just stick in their comfort zone.

If you look at any of the great successful people in life, they have always given up something. Time, not seeing their families, money, eating a restricted diet, no late nights or partying!

For example, during his long career at the top of athletics, Mo Farah spent time away from his family to train at altitude, slept in an oxygen chamber, and restricted his life entirely to: sleep, train and eat; sleep, train and eat. Why? Because he has always been a professional, has wanted to achieve his best... and his results speak for themselves.

Many professional athletes even continue to perform and compete when seriously injured.

Kerri Strug competed on a broken ankle to secure a gold medal for the United States Women's Gymnastics team at the 1996 Olympics.

I've been in this position too and, like Kerri, I knew the show had to go on. A twisted and swollen ankle from performing a tumble of unsprung mats in 2000 was not going to stop me performing in my gymnastic competition. I taped up my ankle, sprayed it with freeze spray, took some pain killers and carried on.

I love ballet and enjoyed dancing 'en pointe' when I was younger. I'd heard that if you bathed your feet in white spirit, it would harden the skin, so every night that's what I did and then slept with my pointe shoes on so my feet would mould to the shoes and the shoes to my feet. I'm not sure how well I slept mind you!

I didn't even mind seeing my ballet tights stuck to my feet with blood when I removed my pointe shoes because the skin on my toes had rubbed away. It didn't stop me from putting them back on again because that was what I wanted to do. I'm not about 'No Pain, No Gain'. I'm about having the mindset to know what you want; being clear on what you enjoy and knowing you will achieve it.

There is an argument that giving things up to get what you desire is necessary to fully appreciate it. However, I never saw my choices as having to give something up. I still don't. If I am given the choice to go out with some of the mums from school for a drink or to go to an aerial silks class, I don't even think about it. It's aerial silks every time and I don't feel I'm missing anything. At 16, I never felt I missed out by not going shopping on a Saturday with friends because I was dancing or training gymnastics. I was doing what I wanted to do.

Interestingly, when doing some research for this chapter on successful athletes and their 'sacrifices', in any information or interviews I read, many of the athletes said the same. They didn't see their choices as being 'sacrifices'. They wanted to achieve their goal. It was important to them.

Look at it in a different way.

Instead of thinking about what you are willing to give up, focus on what you really want to gain.

Flying through the air

If you are 100% committed and want to improve your health and fitness, that desire outweighs everything else. It becomes your choice.

The question then becomes, how much do you want to live a long, active and healthy life? How much do you want to remain fit, strong, mobile and flexible? Do you want it enough?

Do you want it enough to give each and every Pilates workout everything you've got, even when there is no one there saying, "You can do it, one more!"?

Do you want it enough to let go, to let others help you so you can do your Pilates every day?

Do you want it enough to have aching muscles the next day after a workout?

Whilst you ponder on these questions, let me share a story with you.

Ever heard of a free cartwheel or aerial? It's like a cartwheel except you do it in the air without putting your hands down on the floor. Well, I have a video on a VHS tape as proof that I could free cartwheel. However, I couldn't do it for a long time. It was a skill that we needed in our trio routine in order to be scored at the maximum level. My two partners could do it, but not me.

I was so determined. I was 19 and physically capable of doing it, but you find you have a different mentality when you get older. At 8 or 9 years old, I would happily throw myself off people's shoulders onto crash mats, somersault off my partner's wrists, throw myself in the air, because I knew my coaches would catch me and even if I did fall, I would just bounce back up. I did land on my back once on the floor after doing a 'pitch back somersault' and winded myself. I got my breath back, dusted myself off and did the somersault again without thinking twice.

At 19 though, I was more aware that I could injure myself and I really couldn't afford to injure myself as I cycled every day to university training to be a teacher and that would have been problematic if I couldn't get around. I had to get over a huge mental block to just run and throw my head down, throw my arms by my side, kick my legs and defy the laws of gravity to sail through the air and land gracefully back on my feet. Every time I ran up, I wouldn't fully commit! When my coach gave me the minimum required support, I could do it. If my coach stepped away, I couldn't do it. I'd practise from a springboard, I'd practise onto crashmats, off from a higher pile of mats. I'd practise just the step and kick into it, but every time I'd land on my knees or my elbows, or put a hand down, and get cross and frustrated with myself that I was stopping myself from performing it.

How much did I really want to free cartwheel?

Did I want it enough to commit 100%, physically and mentally, and not give up?

I gave up my weekends as a student, Friday and Saturday nights out with friends, evenings which I could have spent with my boyfriend. Actually, if I'm honest, I'd always spent evenings and weekends training, and I didn't drink alcohol because it affected my training. I was so committed to being able to achieve a free cartwheel, that desire outweighed everything else at the time.

So, I *was* committed 100% and the day I finally did it, by committing mentally, believing in myself, visualising the movement, and just going for it – it felt easy! And once I'd done it once, I'd do it everywhere, and loved the feeling that, even at 19, I could still achieve new skills in gymnastics. It just felt so good to fly through the air, be momentarily weightless and land neatly and then stretch, hold my head up high as if to say, "There, easy, I knew I could do it!"

Achieving this meant we could enter our routine with a higher starting score and have a better chance of winning the next competition. I had gained better mental strength, improved my self-esteem and felt very proud. I said I was going to do it and I did! I couldn't have achieved it on my own, though. My coach's and partners' support, encouragement and accountability were essential to my success.

There are no short cuts to good health

Another way to look at this is to flip it on its head. Instead of asking, what are you willing to give up to keep healthy, fit, strong and flexible, we could ask what are you willing to give up if you **don't** keep healthy, fit, strong and flexible?

What are you preventing yourself from gaining if you don't let go of some of your short-term pleasures?

Just think about that for a moment.

My husband is an osteopath and together we run an osteopathic practice. The majority of people who visit our practice are people in pain. This means they have got to the end of the road, perhaps not listened to their body along the way, and certainly not moved enough or in a balanced way. They have often neglected their health and fitness, and then visit the practice, pass the responsibility of their health onto my husband and expect him to work a miracle, in just one visit, even though the problem will have been building up for years.

Patients say, "Can you just sort the problem?" or "I need it sorted before I go on holiday next week."

As professionals we both know it takes time for the body to heal, rebalance and start to move better. Patients will focus on the pain and believe that once the pain has gone, the problem is solved. We explain that we don't treat pain (the symptom) – instead, we look to improve the movement and function, and find the cause of the problem.

My husband and I work together to provide care plans which involve a combination of osteopathic manipulation and Pilates. This has proved to be extremely successful because the osteopathy can improve movement in joints that have become so fixed that it requires expert manual manipulation to release, and then Pilates gives the patient back their responsibility and ownership of their health, builds strength, improves flexibility and rebalances their posture. Both approaches complement each other and enable people to move better. We are about improving functional movement.

Your health is your responsibility but unless you want to improve, and I mean really want to improve how you move so you can do all those things you enjoy doing, then it won't happen.

By the way, my husband is an expert technician when it comes to manual manipulation. He has spoken nationally and internationally to other osteopaths and healthcare practitioners and is sought out by osteopaths in the UK and abroad who want to learn from him how to effectively perform manual manipulation because they haven't learnt it during their training. Check out his YouTube channel and our practice by searching 'Alma Osteopathic Practice' at YouTube.com.

Movement is Life

What happens if you don't move? If you slow down and stop moving?

What do people always say happens if you retire and just sit at home? You gradually just fade away.

I am very fortunate to have a grandmother who has reached 100 years old and still lives independently on her own and we all joke that she has got to that age because she is so stubborn. She likes to do everything herself. A few years ago, the post arrived through the letterbox whilst I was there and I said, "I'll pick it up for you Nan".

She replied, "No, I'll do it. If I don't keep doing it, then I won't be able to do it."

At 100 she still gets herself up and dressed and has breakfast, because she's not waiting for the carers to arrive at 11.00am to do it, as by then it would almost be lunchtime and she'd be hungry!

When we stop moving, our circulation slows, we can get cold, we can gain weight, feel tired and lethargic, as we are taking in less oxygen. Our muscles are not used so grow weak, our joints aren't used and grow stiff, our spine compresses and our posture collapses as gravity's force takes its toll on our body. We then struggle to get up out of a chair, walk upstairs, put our socks and shoes on, get out in the fresh air, carry groceries, and stand and cook lifting heavy pans.

This can all add up and lead to more serious physical health conditions such as heart disease, type 2 diabetes and cardiovascular problems. We are more prone to falls and injuries and our bodies take longer to heal. (www.who.int/health-topics/ physical-activity and www.nhs.uk/live-well/exercise/)

It also leads to the often-unseen conditions such as reduced confidence, loneliness, anxiety, depression, poor sleep and other mental health problems. (Martinsen (2009) and www.sleepfoundation.org/insomnia/exercise-and-insomnia)

Research demonstrates that remaining physically active keeps our body and mind young and healthy. (www.sciencedaily.com/releases/2018/03/180308143123.htm and Gries, K et al (2018))

Joseph Pilates also observed how our age is determined by how much we move.

> *'You are only as young as your spine is flexible.*
> *If your spine is inflexibly stiff at*
> *30, you are old. If it is completely*
> *flexible at 60, you are young'*
>
> Pilates (1945, p16)

Movement is life. When we don't move, we are not allowing ourselves to enjoy the most independent, active and healthy life that is available to us.

So, my question remains – do you want to live a long, active, independent and healthy life enough?

Instant gratification – how effective is it for us?

It may seem difficult to really visualise that far in the future, to us being much older, especially when our day-to-day lives take over and we become more concerned with everything we have to do right now and we're not thinking about our lives in the future.

As human beings we want to see results immediately.

We are flawed by nature. Our ancient ancestors had to chase immediate rewards just to survive. They needed to move to keep warm and find food, they needed to eat food if it was available and to rest to conserve energy. Lieberman (2021)

We seek the instant reward, the bikini body in just 4 weeks, the 6-pack in 21 days, the pain in our backs to disappear instantly, the glass of wine after a hectic day, the tin of biscuits to lift our mood, the TV to allow our mind and body to rest.

How long does that gratification last for? Is it worth giving up our long-term health for?

Do you end up giving up on exercising because you let other pressures take over? Is your exercise the first thing that goes when your schedule gets busy? Does it drop off the end of your To Do list? Or feels like another chore you need to do or should do?

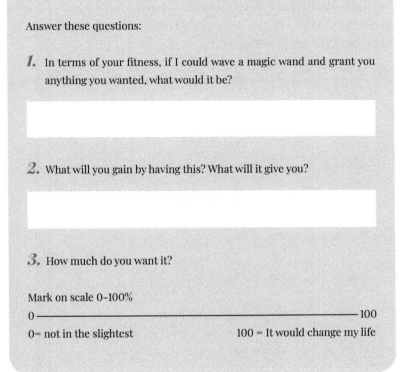

Get Thinking

Answer these questions:

1. In terms of your fitness, if I could wave a magic wand and grant you anything you wanted, what would it be?

2. What will you gain by having this? What will it give you?

3. How much do you want it?

Mark on scale 0-100%

0 ———————————————————————————— 100

0= not in the slightest   100 = It would change my life

You don't have to be Mo Farah.

Focus on what you want to gain, how you will benefit and then it becomes your choice.

Tangible benefits may not materialise before our eyes, but they build up, inevitably manifesting in all manner of ways. If future gains are too far away, then focus on the immediate payoff: feeling fabulous after your Pilates session, because you've kept your self-integrity and taken positive action to keep your body moving.

Now, I'm not suggesting you must live like Mo Farah or carry on struggling through injuries. However, it's about having the mindset of a healthy, fit and strong woman who lives a healthy, active life. Stick with this for at least 80% of the time and you'll be good. You can still have an indulgent meal out and eat what you fancy or take an evening off to watch a film with your kids, but then you're back on with it the next day without beating yourself up about it. (Matthews (2018))

Who you are will make all the difference and this is what I'm going to talk about in the coming chapters.

So, before we continue, I'd like you to make your commitment.

My Commitment

I _____ (your name) am 100% committed to improving my health and fitness.

I am going to read this book, answering the questions, doing the thinking, completing the tasks and get up and get moving to the best of my ability. I'm not going to overthink it or become overwhelmed.

My choice is to enjoy this process and my journey of transformation.

I choose to do this for myself.
I am giving myself permission.
I want this enough.

Signed: _____

Date: _____

Chapter 3

Think, Be, Move

Dreaming of aerial silks

Have you ever seen the Moscow State Circus?

If you haven't then I would highly recommend it.

If you have, you'll have seen the beautiful acrobats that perform graceful, flowing skills of strength and flexibility on just two pieces of silk fabric that hang from the ceiling.

I've watched aerial silk artists perform several times and always thought how much I'd love to be able to do that. It looks absolutely amazing.

But I never did anything about it. Where would I go to learn it? I'd have to travel to London probably, which is too far, and I didn't want to join the circus – I just wanted to have a go.

So, when I turned 40 years old, I decided to investigate and, would you believe it, there was an aerial silks class only a 15-minute drive from me. I signed up for a beginner's course and now, 5 years later, I go to a class or a 1-to-1 session almost every week.

And you know what, I love it just as much as I thought I would, even though I'm twice the age of everyone else in the class. Even though there are days when I try a new skill that the instructor shows me, thinking that looks easy, I can do that, and then discover that in reality it is not as easy as she made it look. Even though my back doesn't bend as much as it used to. Even though I'm the only one not taking a photo of myself to post on my Instagram page. Even though there are days when I can't seem to do anything I'd been able to do the week before!

Then I remind myself that I'm 45 years old and I'm not only keeping up with the 20-year-old girls, but quite often surprise myself when I can do something they are struggling with, when I'm quietly still doing the conditioning and I look around and they've all collapsed on the floor! It's a wonderfully supportive environment, everyone encouraging and bringing out the best in each other.

All that is not just down to the strength in my body, from Pilates, it's down to the strength in my mind. If I didn't have a strong mental approach, I would have arrived at that first class and told myself that I was too old, there was no way I could do it, I'll end up making a fool of myself, and I'd have walked straight back out again and gone home, feeling rubbish about myself.

Aerial silks is not easy. At the studio where I train, everyone has respect for the silks. Performing on other aerial equipment is one thing, but when performing aerial silks, you really need to be able to defy the laws of gravity – you are climbing up silk fabric – it's slippery!!! You need enough strength to get into a move AND enough strength to get back out of it again, otherwise you are just a hanging mess in the air, and you are stuck!

Every time I train, I leave with forearms pumped up, bruises on my thighs and feet, and you never want to experience a silk burn – like a carpet burn but on more delicate areas of your body! Ouch!

I remember when I first started, thinking that I really needed to have more strength so I could learn the technique of each move, but I also needed to be able to perform the technique so I could build the strength I needed to execute it easily. You need both strength and technique.

The only way I've achieved this is by continuing to practise. Continuing to protect my time to go and train consistently – even if that means my husband looks after all the children whilst one of them has their swimming lesson. Even if it means I pick my daughter up from dancing, drop her back home to be with my husband and head straight back out again, leaving my husband to do bedtime. Even if it means scheduling my work hours around studio time. Currently, a Tuesday night is my night to go to my silks class. It's non-negotiable!

That might seem a bit harsh or selfish – and if I'm honest with you, a few years ago, I would have thought the same.

What's wrong with me?

There was a period in my life, when my children were all little, when I didn't do any 'exercise'.

For 30 years previously, being physically active had just been an integral part of my life. I'd never questioned it. It was such a big part of my life that I even did it as a job. My specialism in my teaching degree was physical education. I later became a Physical Education Consultant, coached sports acrobatics gymnastics and trampolining, became a Pilates teacher and did a dissertation and further research on movement.

So, I thought, it must be me. Something was wrong with ME. How could other women appear to work, look after children, and be fit and healthy but I was struggling, especially when only 4 years previously, being active and moving was all I did?

I thought my problem was that I didn't have enough time – more on that later.

Actually, the reason I wasn't doing any exercise or activity *was* to do with me. It wasn't that there was anything 'wrong' with me and there is nothing 'wrong' with you if you are feeling the same.

As women we have lots of behaviours and beliefs that are deep in our evolution (nature) and that we inherit from society (nurture) that are held in high regard by others, but that actually don't benefit us. I'll come back to this point too.

After several years of berating myself over my lack of exercise I discovered the secret to fitness success for busy women – and it's simple:

There are just 3 elements that make up my unique approach to fitness for when you are a busy woman with a career and a family:

1. Think
2. Be
3. Move

These 3 parts make up your Triangle of Strength.

The Triangle of Strength

A triangle is the strongest shape, but for it to be successful and not collapse, it needs all 3 sides to be connected.

This is the same for you to be your best self – if one of the three elements is missing, you'll just make it harder for yourself.

It requires a strong mind, strong behaviours and a strong, effective way of moving to be a fit, active and healthy woman. To be living as your Best Empowered Self.

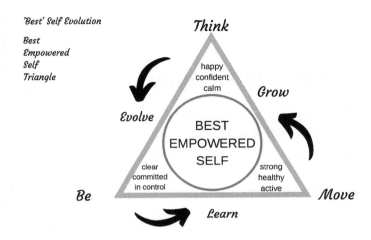

'Best' Self Evolution

Best
Empowered
Self
Triangle

Another way to think of it is that you need three types of strength: mental strength, behavioural strength and physical strength.

What do I mean by strength?

The Oxford Dictionary definition is:

1. the quality or state of being physically strong.
2. the capacity of an object or substance to withstand great force or pressure.

This is not the full definition of strength as I see it. Strength can take different forms.

Let's take each one in turn.

Think strong:
The strength of your mind

For me, having strength of mind is about knowing you have a choice. You can choose how to live your life. Choose who to be and make decisions that benefit you. You are at peace with your choices. You feel happy, confident and calm.

Let me give you an example of what I mean.

"Go on then, Miss Parris," (that was my maiden name) "show us how to do it!"

I was in the middle of teaching a Year 8 boys' gymnastics lesson (13-year-old boys!) and we were doing vaulting – where you run, jump on a springboard, and fly over a box/horse.

I was 29 years old at the time and had retired from gymnastics several years previously.

I was teaching the boys fly spring, where the box is length ways, you run up, jump on the springboard, reach for the furthest end of the box with your hands, straddle your legs around the side to bring them in front of you at the same time as pushing off the box and landing neatly on two feet on the landing mat.

So, when the boys asked me to show them what to do, I hesitated, and several thoughts ran through my mind.

"OK," I said to myself, "this could go one of two ways. I am either going to do it, go for it, hope my body and brain remember what they are doing and if I'm lucky I'll make it unscathed to the mats, make out it was just like a walk in the park and simultaneously become the coolest teacher in school, with automatic respect from the children..."

OR

"I can have a go and could not make it, land with my legs either side of the box in a somewhat painful position, or bang my coccyx, miss my landing, my feet disappear from underneath me and I fall flat on my face, with a worst-case scenario of the children running to the office to get first aid and even a trip to the hospital."

I had to make a decision, with all the Year 8 boys looking at me, probably some willing for the latter scenario to unfold.

Of course, there was a third option, which was say, "No, I can't do it", but for me that wasn't an option, that was just giving up and admitting to myself I couldn't do it, without even trying. If I didn't do it, I'd be cross with myself for not even trying. So no, I was going to do it.

Now, with vaulting, you need to commit 100%. You can't do it in a half-hearted way – because that's exactly how you will injury yourself. You have to go for it. I have on so many occasions in my training run up to the vault to just slow down before reaching the box and ended up turning round to start again.

Physically, I knew I would be OK, even if I was going to be a bit sore the next day. Mentally, I had to believe I could do it. I had to stand there, see the vault in front of me and visualise doing it. Visualise achieving it and becoming the coolest teacher ever! Visualise doing it easily and showing the boys that if I could do it, they could too.

I needed my physical strength, but I really needed my mental strength too.

You'll be pleased to hear that I became the coolest teacher in school and had respect from the coolest Year 8 boys. Of course, they then wanted to achieve it too!

If I had doubted myself, started overthinking it and talking myself out of it, I fear it would not have been a pretty sight. And even to this day, I'm so pleased with myself that I just did it, I made that commitment to myself.

You might think, well that's fine for me, if you've been a gymnast before, that was no big thing. But it doesn't matter how many times I have stood at the edge of the mat before walking on to compete or stood backstage before a dance performance, I would always and still do feel nervous.

In gymnastics competitions when you are nervous, and the palms of hands go clammy and your feet sweaty, it really doesn't help when you then have to hold a balance. There was always one balance my trio were hit and miss with. It was the 'three high' – one on top of the next person's shoulders. By the way, a trick we would do before competing was to spray our thighs with hairspray, so they were sticky when our partner stood on them, and this stopped them slipping as they climbed up onto shoulders! I don't think it made any difference scientifically, but we believed it did – and that was all that mattered!

You had to hold it for a minimum of 3 seconds once you were in place for it to be judged. If you fall out at 2.5 seconds, you've lost the mark and, the reality was, if you dropped a balance, you were out of the competition. Unless of course everyone else did too!

I can remember times when we dropped balances – and we knew that was the competition over – but you couldn't just walk off the mats or stamp your feet or cry or doing anything else you felt like doing, you carried on. That's just what you did. You remained professional and kept a strength of mind to hold the remainder of the routine together so you could finish with some dignity. I was always at peace with the choices I made as a competitive gymnast, even if we didn't perform as well as we knew we could.

The voice in your head

However, having the strength of mind in the situations I've described above was easy in comparison to when I became a mum. It is only recently that I have really understood how I was sabotaging my own efforts to be active and why, and how unkind I was to myself.

In 2015, my children were 1, 2 and 4 years old. I knew I wanted to start to get back in shape and feel good about myself.

So, I found a ballet class to go to. It was a 30-minute drive away and I had to find somewhere to park when I got there. It was an evening class, 7.30–8.30pm.

I'd book and pay for the class, make sure my husband could look after the children and then spend all day finding 'reasons' why I couldn't go. I'd have these draining conversations with myself about how really I needed to do the finances for my husband's business at the end of the day before I went, that really I should be the one to read a bedtime story, that I should really stay at home and look after the children so my husband could do his training. Which, by the way, he never misses, ever. In the whole 25 years I've known him, he *never* misses his training.

By the time I needed to leave, I was mentally exhausted from ruminating over 'should I go or not' all day, that I would then decide I was too tired, and I'd just try and go next week. I would then beat myself up about not going and start another conversation with myself about how I should have gone, no one was stopping me, resenting my husband because he always got to do his training and I felt I never got a chance to exercise.

I believed all my excuses were justified reasons and I told myself so often that I didn't see what I was doing, and it just became my reality.

Maybe this sounds familiar, and you have similar conversations with yourself?

Well, let me reassure you that I very rarely have these conversations with myself anymore and even if that little voice sometimes rears its head, it's much quieter these days, as I know how to ignore it.

And it feels so good!

Stay with me and I'll share my experiences and how I have developed a strong mind so you too can ignore that other voice in your head.

Get Moving

Take your left ear to your left shoulder, then right ear to right shoulder, repeat. Turn your head right and left, looking over each shoulder in turn, nod your head down, chin to chest, lift and look up at the ceiling.

Roll your shoulders backwards 4 times, then the elbows, making the circles bigger each time, and then circle the arms back 4 times. Reverse, starting with the shoulders and taking them forward, again 4 times for each.

Circle one arm back and the other arm forward at the same time 4 times (this is a bit like patting your head and rubbing your tummy – it takes brain power – but don't over-think it.) Then reverse and change direction for each arm 4 times.

Did you do it?

Feel better?

Be strong:
Strength in how you are being

This is the second strength I want to talk about. Strength in how you are being I would describe as making choices about who you are and how you want to be, creating habits and actions that align with your being and that serve you.

We have a choice about which thoughts to focus on and we have a choice in how we respond in different situations.

As Jen Sincero (2013) explains, our thinking eventually becomes our reality.

'Our thoughts become our words
Our words become our beliefs
Our beliefs become our actions
Our actions become our habits
Our habits become our realities'

Jen Sincero

If we focus on the thoughts that do not benefit us, then it's also the case that our habits and actions will not benefit us either.

For example, you think of yourself as a fit, active woman with plenty of time to exercise, your behaviours follow. They become automatic, habits that serve us.

We are physically active. We don't think about it, we don't have long debates with ourselves about it, we don't find excuses not to do it, it just happens easily and is part of us and our lifestyle.

Just like brushing your teeth. You don't get up each morning and decide whether to brush your teeth or not. You just do it, because you're the sort of woman who has clean teeth.

It makes no difference if it's raining, it's Monday morning or Saturday night, if you've had a bad day or feel tired. You just do it – because it is a habit, a strong way of being, a part of who you are.

It is also about making decisions and following through on them, keeping your self-integrity. Every time you break a promise to yourself you damage your self-esteem. You value yourself a little less.

Earlier in this chapter, I mentioned to you that my aerial silks class on a Tuesday was non-negotiable. Well, you know what I am only human and, on my journey, too.

Here's what happened...

As you know, I had been going to my aerial silks class on a Tuesday night. I'd been going every week and going consistently.

Then my eldest son's swimming lesson changed and guess when it changed to? Yes, exactly the same time as my silks class.

So, what did I do? I immediately said, yes that's fine he can go swimming and I'll miss silks and try and do a private session instead.

What happened? I took my son swimming, whilst my husband stayed at home with my youngest two children and put them to bed. The swimming lesson was fairly late and past my youngest son and daughter's bedtime.

Did I do any 1-to-1 sessions? Yes, I did one... in about 3 months! Not regularly enough to maintain my strength.

Then a few months later, my youngest son's swimming lesson changed to a Tuesday night too – slightly earlier. It made sense for me to take both boys to swimming together and get my youngest changed whilst my eldest was still swimming. My husband stayed at home so my daughter could get to bed.

Now, my daughter is a night owl, is often awake late and enjoys a lie-in in the mornings. I'd get home from taking the boys to their swimming lesson and she would still be awake.

It may seem obvious to you reading this now, but at the time I didn't see it straight away. However, I'm not beating myself up about it, because several years earlier that would have been the end of the story and the end of me going to silks. I would have waited until swimming lessons changed time again and then maybe have gone back to it. In the meantime, feeling resentful that everyone else was doing their activities except me. Even as I write that, it doesn't feel good – but I'm being honest. That's how I would have felt. I would have dismissed it immediately as being selfish.

However, a couple of weeks later I did see a solution that benefited everyone.

You've guessed it – my husband now takes all three children to swimming, my daughter watches and colours, my boys swim, they come home and get into bed and go to sleep. Meanwhile, I go to silks, come home, say goodnight and have a shower! Everyone is happy, everyone is able to get to the right place at the right time and the children get to do their swimming lesson. My husband gets to spend some individual time with our daughter, and I get to go to my silks class.

Now, there will come a point when the swimming lessons change again and then we will have a new plan. Planning your physical activity is one strong behaviour you need – a Plan A, Plan B and possibly a Plan C too when you are a busy woman, but we will come onto this later, when we dive deeper into a strong way of being.

Move strong:
Strength in your body

This is the third and final strength. Physical strength is closest to the definition in the dictionary and possibly the one that first comes to mind when you think about strength.

For me, though, physical strength is so much more than just lifting heavy weights. It's about holding your body in a good posture, being able to move efficiently and effectively, being able to do everything you enjoy and as you get older remain active and independent.

Physical strength is about control, balance, flow, grace, precision, being centred and aligned and being able to move in a functional, efficient, effortless and effective way.

'Pilates [Contrology] begins with mind control over muscles. It reawakens thousands and thousands of dormant muscle cells and brain cells.'

Pilates (1945, p10)

It's about knowing when to rest and when to keep going. It's about listening to your body and being connected to your body.

Take a bodybuilder or picture one of the world's strongest men – they are stronger than you and I for sure, but their mobility and movement can often appear awkward and restricted. Their arms don't swing by the sides of their body. They walk with their weight shifting side to side because their legs don't swing past each other easily. They often injure themselves, pop a bicep muscle or hamstring because they have the strength in the muscle but not the flexibility. They are muscle-bound.

Now picture a rhythmic gymnast who cannot just bend backwards and touch her head to her toe, but also get her feet behind her and then under her chin, who can hyper-split, with legs going beyond splits. She is flexible, but at what expense? If she doesn't have the strength in her muscles she will only suffer from injuries and long-term damage to her body. People who are hypermobile often suffer from joints dislocating and other injuries. I teach a few women who are hypermobile, and we work on improving their core strength, improving stability in their pelvis and hip joints and in their shoulders.

It is all about achieving a balance between strength and flexibility.

I have to acknowledge that the one physical activity I have continued to do since retiring from gymnastics and dancing, is Pilates. I continued to teach and demonstrate Pilates through each of my three pregnancies and when my children were little. It is Pilates that enables me to still have the core strength and flexibility to do aerial silks and return to ballet at 45 years old.

To gain, maintain and improve your physical strength you have to exercise consistently. Doing HIIT (High Intensity Interval Training) once in the blue moon just doesn't work. You are more likely to injure yourself than build long-term functional strength and fitness. Consistency is key and to be consistent is a strong way of being – it's a habit.

If you are juggling work life and family life though, it is not always easy to remain consistent. If your life is similar to mine, each day is completely different. Each week is different. Now I love this, but it doesn't make it easy when planning in physical activity for yourself.

It's much easier to be able to fit some movement into your schedule rather than having to overhaul your schedule to find time to exercise. As humans we prefer the path of least resistance, so let's make it easy and then it's more likely to happen.
(Clear (2018))

I don't live to 'exercise'. I keep moving and remain physically active so I can live.

Once I had developed a strong mind and strong way of being I was then able to use the knowledge of Pilates and movement and found myself doing a few Pilates moves here, a few stretches there, in between playing with my children, cooking, working etc.

And then I realised that what I was doing was Bitesize Pilates. Pilates sessions broken up into small chunks. Finding 20 minutes of uninterrupted time is easier than finding time to go to a class, plus travel time and the time being imposed on you as to when to go. I was then able to be consistent with my 'exercise' and therefore started feeling stronger again, was moving more easily again, my backache disappeared, and I felt good about myself.

> *'Pilates [Contrology] is not a fatiguing system of dull, boring, abhorred exercises repeated daily ad-nauseum. Neither does it demand your joining a gymnasium nor purchasing of expensive equipment apparatus. You may derive all the benefits of Contrology in your own home.'*
>
> Pilates (1945, p10)

It's all connected

Although I knew how to move and what to do – I had been a gymnastic coach, a trampolining coach, a PE teacher, a PE consultant, and a Pilates teacher, having the knowledge of what to do didn't help me on its own. Even though before I had my children being physically active had been a habit, I'd lost that habit and didn't know how to get it back.

I started 'doing' some of the right things, for example I'd book and pay for an exercise class, make sure my husband could look after the children, had everything in place to go – but more often than not I'd say, "Well, I haven't got enough time to go, so I'll just miss it and go next week."

When I did force myself to go, and I use the word 'force' because that's what it felt like, I'd just keep checking the time, hoping they'd finish the class on time so I could get back home. I wouldn't engage in the class fully because there was a voice in my head that kept telling me I 'should' be at home looking after the children, that I had other responsibilities and it was selfish of me to go out and do something for myself.

I knew how to move – I was still teaching Pilates all through this time – but that was OK because I was doing it for other people and had made a commitment to them. I had certain behaviours in place to allow me to do my 'exercise', such as planning the time, getting childcare etc, BUT... there was still something else that was stopping me.

I had told myself too often that I was too tired, too busy, should clean the house first or do the children's packed lunches, that I started to believe it. I believed that I just didn't have enough time, and this then became my reality. I THOUGHT I couldn't BE a successful mum and a healthy, active woman too. I couldn't BE both.

What finally changed?

ME!

I finally realised that how I was thinking, behaving and moving was my choice.

It was all my choice.

It was not my fault because at the time I didn't know any different.

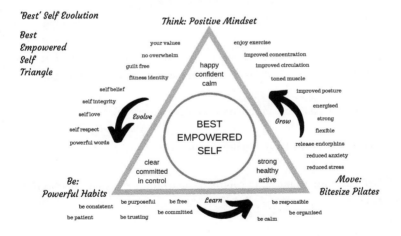

This is a process of gradual change that has taken me 5 years. The brain is like a muscle and takes exercising and practice just like the muscles in the body.

It doesn't happen overnight. You don't go to the gym and come out an hour later with a defined 6-pack. In the same way, you don't read a few positive quotes or attend a mindset workshop and leave with a completely different perspective that sticks.

You may get some shifts in your perspective, a lightbulb moment or enlightenment that starts the chain reaction, but to make it a part of you takes practice.

It's a process that needs reviewing, reflecting on and tweaking as you evolve, learn and grow, and we will take each element in turn in the following chapters.

To become your best empowered self you need the awareness, strategies, tools, and the knowing – deep in your centre, your 'core' – and to enjoy the process and journey of becoming your best empowered self.

Get Thinking

Just take a moment and imagine you are a woman who enjoys leading a physically active and fulfilling life with true strength, confidence and calm...

You have enough time and energy to do Pilates every day.

You build strength, become more flexible and stand taller.

You feel more confident, in control of your fitness and your mind feels clear and calm.

You sleep better and make healthy choices.

How does that feel?

Have you considered that this is possible for you?

It is possible to think, be and move in a way that benefits you – it's your choice.

It's your choice which thoughts you focus on.

It's your choice to be the person you want to be.

It's your choice to do Pilates, so you can feel good mentally and physically.

It took me many years to discover how my thinking and behaviours were not helping me to look after myself in body and mind.

But because you are here, reading this book, you have a head-start.

You've already made a start just by reading this book and you're now already at the end of Chapter 3.

I used to wish that someone could have pointed out to me what I was doing, but then I perhaps wasn't in the right place to hear them if they had said something.

But now, I know that I'm glad I did go through these years of struggle with my fitness because I've learnt so much about myself that I can share with others who I know are likely to feel the same. My experiences can help you and other women like you to make those changes quickly and easily.

Chapter 4

Get out of your own way

*L*et's now look more deeply at your Triangle of Strength, and the first part we will explore is **Think: A Positive Mindset**. I will share with you the same strategies I have used myself and use successfully to help my clients.

Who are you?

If you're going to get out of your own way, then you need to know who you are first, so you know who it is that's getting in your way.

Get Thinking

Write below:

Who you are, as if you were introducing yourself at one of those ice-breaking activities at the start of courses/meetings where you have to go round one by one and state who you are:

Why are you here?

Have you ever felt like you've lost your way? You've lost yourself and who you are?

If you have, you'll understand how I felt several years ago.

As you now know I'd always led an active lifestyle, I didn't know any different. That was who I was. That was Gila. I never questioned it.

> ## *"The person who incorporates exercise into their identity doesn't have to convince themselves to train.'*
>
> Clear (2018, p34)

As I'd grown up, I'd been praised and rewarded for being conscientious and hard-working. I was a gymnast, a dancer, super flexible, strong, fit and active.

That was until I became a mum. I stopped being Gila and became a mum. By the time I'd had my three children, I had left my job as a PE consultant after my second child and stopped any freelance work after my third. I wanted to spend time with my children when they were little, and I was fortunate enough that as a family we had that choice.

My husband's business had been growing and so I happily helped him out by doing some of the behind-the-scenes jobs. This evolved into taking on an HR role and a finance role. Neither of which I really knew how to do, so I learnt on the job, which is quite scary when that involves being responsible for paying someone's salary!

The advantage with this work was it was flexible around looking after my children and of course it helped my husband and ultimately our family.

My eldest started school and I started to meet other mums. Naturally, you chat and start to get to know each other. They would ask me, "What do you do, Gila?"

I'd reply, "I'm a mum of three children and I help my husband in his business."

That was it. This was how I described myself for about 7 years.

People would then say, "Oh, you must be busy then?" or "Wow, how do you do it with three children and working?"

Well, because that's what you do isn't when you become a mum and it's something to be proud of isn't it?

Yes, I was 'busy', I worked hard, I was doing everything for my children, lots of things for my husband, helping at summer fayres, washing, cooking, cleaning, going to swimming lessons, doing payroll, tax returns, training our receptionist on new software, being at the end of the phone if she rang with a query, answering it even if it was teatime, and cashing up at the end of the day often as late as 9.00pm.

So yes, you could say I was busy – I was doing everything for everyone else.

This is the time that I struggled with my fitness and exercise. There was no way I could go to an exercise class with so many responsibilities.

It wasn't until I went on a women's business retreat that the penny dropped, and I started to change my life and my thinking. That was in 2019.

I had really had to convince myself it was OK to go on this business retreat for two days and leave my husband and my children. I'd miss them of course, but I was also struggling to let go of the control of being needed at home to do everything. However, one thing that helped sway me was that my nanna lived near where the retreat was, and I could take the opportunity to see her.

I had arrived at this remote, rural setting with its several converted barns, that looked luxurious, had hot tubs, tea and coffee available on arrival, not knowing anyone and feeling very out of my depth surrounded by successful businesswomen.

I was assigned a beautiful room, with king-size bed and ensuite, overlooking the fields.

The retreat started and we all had to introduce ourselves and say why we were there.

So, when it came to my turn, I said, "Hi, I'm Gila, I have three children and I'm here to help my husband grow his business."

"Thank you, Gila. But tell me why you are here."

I was confused. Why had the business mentor leading this retreat just repeated the question? I'd just said why I was there. Hadn't she heard me?

I replied again: "I am here so I can help my husband grow his business."

"No," she said. "Why are YOU here?"

Thanks to Jo Davison – Blue Cow and womanpreneur – she was the first person in a long time who had told me what I needed to hear.

I didn't know what to say. I felt embarrassed. Why was 'I' there? I really couldn't answer, because it had been such a long time that I had thought about myself.

You see, I had this belief that you couldn't be a successful mum *and* a successful woman in business at the same time. It was one or the other.

The point of telling you this story is that my identity was defined by my role in relation to others. I'd lost my 'own' identity, so I didn't know what was important to me. I was saying unhelpful things to myself and, let's be honest, just making excuses, which at the time I saw as justified reasons!

Our identity can have a direct impact on how we see exercise.

Take a look at the following and see if you relate to any or a few of these identities that I have come across in myself and in the women I've worked with.

What is your Fitness Identity?

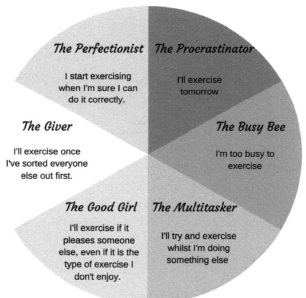

The Perfectionist
I start exercising when I'm sure I can do it correctly.

The Procrastinator
I'll exercise tomorrow

The Giver
I'll exercise once I've sorted everyone else out first.

The Busy Bee
I'm too busy to exercise

The Good Girl
I'll exercise if it pleases someone else, even if it is the type of exercise I don't enjoy.

The Multitasker
I'll try and exercise whilst I'm doing something else

Get Thinking

Write down which identities you relate to most. It can be more than one.

In the past I was definitely the 'busy bee, the multitasker and the giver' but this identity was not helping me to exercise.

Who are you expected to be?

Expectations come from ourselves, from others and from society. Expectations of women are often different than those of men, and the expectations we hold are reflected in how we behave, what we value, and these don't always benefit us.

'In many ways, these social norms are the invisible rules that guide your behaviour each day.' Clear (2018, p115)

The Multitasker

Women can multitask, right?

This has become an accepted belief among most of society and is often held as a badge of honour.

Sometimes, multitasking is unavoidable, and you could argue doesn't have a detrimental effect on what we do. You may have found yourself cooking and having a conversation at the same time or going for a walk and listening to a podcast. If one of the things you are doing you can do on autopilot, like walking, then your brain is free to listen to the podcast and it's no problem. The problem comes when the two or more tasks require the same part of the brain, or we need to consciously think about them.

When we multitask, using the same parts of our brain, it can take longer, more energy and we often make mistakes. For example, have you ever tried to reply to a text message or email at the same time as listening to someone talking to you? Both use words and so you lose your train of thought, and you end up not really listening to what the person is saying and having to keep re-reading what you've written. Your brain is having to continually switch tasks, which is mentally draining.

I'd like you to try something for me to demonstrate this.

Get Thinking

Get a piece of paper and pen.

Set a timer and write the first letter of the alphabet, followed by the number 1, followed by number 1 as a roman numeral. Underneath that, write the next letter, number, roman numeral and so on up to 26, and then stop the timer.

e.g.
A 1 I
B 2 II
C 3 III

D 4 IV

Etc.

Write down how long it took you.

Now, set a timer and write down in one column all the letters of the alphabet, first A–Z

A

B

C

D

Etc

Next in a second column write down all the numbers, 1-26

A 1

B 2

C 3

D 4

Thirdly, in a third column write down all the roman numerals, 1-26.

Stop the timer.

Write down how long it took you.

How did you brain feel doing it? Which felt harder?

Although we can't always get away from multitasking, it is not an efficient use of our time. If you are switching tasks all day long and juggling lots of different things, you will feel more mentally exhausted by the end of the day and therefore less like doing any exercise. You are programmed to conserve energy and so your brain will be willing you to rest.

Think about how you work during the day and start to be aware of times when you are multitasking and ask yourself if you could do one thing first and then the next thing. Learning the skill of monotasking has been hugely helpful to me. I don't do it all the time, so I still catch myself at a times, but having this awareness will help you concentrate and leave you with enough mental energy and brain power to still want to exercise.

The Busy Bee

I was at Tesco, collecting my food shopping early in the morning, as I do every week, and the Tesco employee was making polite conversation with me.

"So, have you got a busy day planned?"

"Oh, yes! Always busy!" I replied.

"Well, it's good to keep busy!" he said.

The word 'busy' is used a lot! Just over the next few days, listen out for it in conversations, maybe in what you say in your head or out loud.

These are some of things I hear:

"If you want something done, always ask a busy person."

This was true in my first teaching position. People knew I was busy, I was proud of this fact, and so they'd ask me to do more, and I'd say yes and continue to be busy.

"Hi, how are you?"

"Good, thank you, busy, but good."

Ever had a similar conversation?

I used to say this all the time too, it was my default reply. As if I needed to qualify and justify my existence. Notice the 'but'. Being busy was not necessarily 'good' but it was something to say that told other people to expect less of me and simultaneously showing that I had a purpose, I had everything under control.

"I'm just too busy to do any exercise."

Yep! Something else I used to say.

I had the belief that being busy was a sign of being successful, whether as a teacher, a mum or as a person. But there is being busy and there is being productive.

What I never used to understand was how I was always so busy, but I'd get to the end of the day and say to my husband, "I don't feel like I've achieved anything today".

What on earth was I spending my time doing? I was 'being busy'. And as the definition explains, 'busy' means 'having a great deal to do' and 'keeping oneself occupied'. Neither of which imply achieving anything.

Again, my expectation was not helping me.

Until, a few years ago, a business mentor of mine said,

"You will always be busy until you commit to NOT being busy."

Read that again.

I had committed my life to being busy, working hard and to keep doing.

I was focused on doing, doing, doing and this left me feeling overwhelmed, mentally drained and frustrated, so much so that I never seemed to have time to do anything for myself.

The word 'busy' is just a poor excuse for not making choices and taking responsibility in your life.

So, I make a commitment to NOT be busy anymore. I am now committed to being productive, choosing to invest my time doing things that are important to me and align with my values. I feel so much better for it... and am never too busy to exercise, because my health and fitness is one of my most important values.

The Giver

Get Thinking

Rate your self-care routine 0-10. 0 = non-existent, 10 = perfect, couldn't be better.

0 ————————————————————————————— 10

Going right back to our ancestors, the female has always held a nurturing and caring role, looking after the young of the family.

Women today are often, though not always, in nurturing roles such as nursing, teaching, caring, childminding etc and in these roles we look after everyone else.

But by looking after everyone else, this doesn't mean we can't and shouldn't look after ourselves. You can only pour from a full cup, as the saying goes.

Self-care is not a luxury, a one-off and nor is it selfish. Our own self-care is an essential, daily habit which can happen if we only give ourselves permission.

Because, let's face it, if we don't look after ourselves, who will? Our self-care, our health and fitness are our responsibility.

I always told myself that I'd get everything else done first for everyone else and when it was all done, then I'd allow myself to do my Pilates or go to ballet.

But guess what happened?

I never got to the point when everything was done! So, I never got to do any exercise.

So yet again, this deep instinct to help, nurture and care for others doesn't always benefit us, if we let it stop us from looking after ourselves.

If you identify as a giver, then you too may feel that you can only do your exercise as a reward, when you have done everything else first.

As I said at the start of this book, we all are born with the right to move. It is your right to move, to remain strong and flexible, active and independent because only then will you be in a position to be able to help others.

The Perfectionist

'Practice makes perfect' is a saying I'm sure you've heard but is one that is not true.

If you are aiming to be perfect, let me just tell you now, that perfection doesn't exist. It will save you a lot of time and heartache.

The trouble is, we are bombarded by social media, TV and films with society's expectations of how we should look, how we should behave, what we should do, and these images and expectations are held as the ultimate achievement.

Why do we want to look like someone else? Are you not enough as you are?

Does aiming for perfection stop you from ever starting? I've had women say to me that they didn't want to come to a class because they wouldn't know what to do and wouldn't be able to perform the moves.

No one will perform them perfectly because there is no such thing. You can only perform them as well as you can and you will improve, but you must start.

If you are a perfectionist, does it get in your way of exercising?

The Good Girl

We are conditioned as we grow up to be 'good girls', put our hand up in class and do as we are asked.

Were you a good girl growing up? I was. I wanted to please others.

As I became an adult, I would say yes to things which I didn't really want to do but felt it was what was expected of me.

Maybe for you, the only exercise you do is, for example, to go running with your friend, because you want to be a good friend and support them, even though you really don't enjoy running.

Doing what is important to you – is not being selfish, it is not being a bad girl. It's about having integrity, self-worth and self-respect.

The Procrastinator

Have you ever procrastinated about doing exercise?

Yes – me too!

I never thought I was a procrastinator. I always prided myself in getting things done. The truth is we all procrastinate over something and it's usually the things we don't enjoy doing, but I've found I can procrastinate on things I enjoy doing too. I sometimes enjoy the feeling of looking forward to doing something more than actually doing it, so continue to put it off.

It's easy to get distracted. A message can come up on my phone and then before I realise it 20 minutes has passed and I've ended up finding myself looking at someone's profile that I used to go to school with, comparing my life to the online, unrealistic snapshot of theirs.

What have I achieved? Nothing – apart from feeling annoyed with myself for wasting time and comparing myself to others (never a productive pastime). My reward? I've kept myself in my comfort zone, procrastinating from the task in hand.

You may procrastinate with exercising by saying to yourself, "I'll go for a run when it's stopped raining" or "I'll start going to the gym in the New Year".

However, if we are being purposeful and living in alignment with our values and making decisions that match our values the only procrastinating we need to do is procrastinating on purpose.

By that I mean deciding on purpose that you will leave something to a later time because other things are more important to you.

The difference is, you've made the decision to procrastinate on it.

Get Thinking

Catch yourself procrastinating on your exercise?

Write down, what did you say?

Why did you say it?

What reward are you getting for saying these things and not exercising?

The expectations we've explored above of who you should be were never yours to meet. If they are not serving you, then discard them.

Get Thinking

What expectations do you have that are either your own, or you've adopted from family, growing up, from society, social media or others?

Where have they come from?

Are they true?

Your Values

Deciding what is important to you will give you the freedom from trying to do everything.

What is important to you?

There is a long list you may be choosing from! Here are some words which may prompt you: family, career, health, fitness, friends, experiences, success, money, wealth, food, love, freedom, truth, honesty, achievement, co-operation, exercise, enjoyment, experiences, business, career, fun, discipline, education, potential, independence, helping others, respect, nature, imagination, self-integrity, nurture, social life, laughter, physical activity, loyalty, professionalism, survival, teamwork.

Get Thinking

Write down what is important to you. Choose 10 top things – they can be from my examples above or you can use your own, or a mixture of both. Write each one on a separate Post-it note.

Order them 1-10: 1 = most important, 10 = least important.

Where does your health or fitness come? Is it in the top 5?

I'm assuming it probably is because you are here reading this book.

My highest value has always been my family. Nothing was ever too much trouble – anyone in my family having a problem, no worries, I'd sort it! I'd take it on, do it, wash it, clean it, organise it, mend it, bandage it, feel it, be responsible for it, spend my time on it, spend my energy on it, make it better – no problem!

What I didn't see at the time was how this was driving my actions but was not serving ME! I had not made a conscious decision about what was important to me.

This resulted in me feeling resentful, frustrated, guilty and angry. I blamed everyone else for my lack of time and energy to do anything for me, but actually, I had created that situation myself and had not taken any responsibility for myself and my health and fitness.

My highest value *is* still my family, but I am also clear on what else is important to me and honour that by taking responsibility in those areas of my life. As a result, I am calmer, more relaxed, and at peace with the decisions I make.

You will always find time to do what is important to you, and because I have made a conscious decision that my health and fitness is important to me, I have plenty of time for it.

Being clear on your values will give you a strong foundation on which to base your daily decisions and drive your actions so you can live in alignment with what is important to you.

For example, I know if I need to choose between doing Pilates, ballet or silks and going to the pub for a drink, it's a no brainer. I know exactly what my decision would be, and I am happy with that. I don't feel guilty or spend all day ruminating over my decision. It's done. Living on purpose in this way is liberating, energising and uplifting.

Get Moving

I have a sock challenge for you.

Stand up, remove your shoes/slippers and socks.

Now, armed with one sock, see if you can stand on one leg, lift the other knee up and place your sock over your foot. The aim is to do it without falling over or having to lean on something or cross your sock ankle over your supporting leg. This is a functional movement that you can do every morning when you put your socks on and will not take up any more of your time but will improve your balance and leg strength.

How did you get on?

Now try with the other leg. Was one leg easier than the other?

The power of your words

A wonderful friend and business colleague, Tulay Massey, spoke to my members in 'CORE' (my online Pilates membership for busy women) about the power of our words.

She asked us to close our eyes and move our right arm out to the side and behind us as far as it would go. As we were doing this she was talking and telling us that it was easy, that our arms were light and fluid and it was easy, easy, easy. We then opened our eyes and took a look at how far behind us we had reached.

Then we repeated the exercise, but this time as we moved our arm, Tulay told us it was really hard, that we were struggling to move our arm, it was heavy and restricted, it was really difficult. Then we opened our eyes again to see how far behind us we had reached.

I was amazed at the difference. The second time, when I tried to move my arm, I did feel I just couldn't go any further and it felt much harder than the first time. The difference in how far my arm reached was remarkable. When my brain thought it was easy, I had reached diagonally behind me, but when I thought it was hard, my arm was only out to the side.

Try it yourself if you like by asking someone to speak as Tulay did – it is a great demonstration of the power of our words on our thoughts and actions.

We spend most of our time having conversations with ourselves, and so what we say to ourselves has a huge impact on our thoughts, behaviours, actions and habits.

Have you ever looked in the mirror and said to yourself, "Hey, you are looking fabulous today girl"?

Conversely, have you ever looked in the mirror and said to yourself, "Oh, you could do with losing a bit of weight, you've got bags under your eyes, and those leggings are really not flattering"?

You may have said both. Which do you say most often?

Which would you say to your best friend or sister or daughter?

Certainly not the second example – these are unkind things to say to anyone, including yourself.

I have a pink, glittery sign by my bedside table that I see every morning when I get up that says, 'You are Awesome'. We all need reminding at times and with practice it will become a good habit.

So, in case you need to hear this today:

'You are Awesome'.

You get to choose

How many times have you said to yourself, "I'll try and fit in some exercise today" or "Hopefully I'll get to my exercise class today" or "I'm aiming to do my exercise after tea" or "I know I should do more exercise but..."

I used to say all these things almost every day when my children were little.

The words 'try' and 'hope' and 'aim' are words that show you are not really committed to doing it.

As Yoda says, "Do or do not, there is no try".

Try putting this book down. Did you do it? Well, either you are still holding it or you put it down – there is no in-between.

'Should' is such a heavy word, filled with expectation. We 'should' do exercise, we 'should' go on a walk. Who says you should? Why? How does it make you feel?

The problem with the word 'should' is that it can make everything feel like a chore. You are doing things under duress, and where there is an expectation attached, guilt will follow if we don't meet that expectation.

Remember, it's your choice. You don't have to do any exercise if you don't want to.

Another phrase you might use is 'I can't do this' or 'I'm no good at it'.

But were you ever told as a child, "There is no such thing as can't"?

'Can't' is a word that limits your beliefs. It is final. If you can't do it now, then what's the point in trying?

Think of when you learnt a new skill such as riding a bike. How many times did you fall off and how many times did you get back on and practise? Then you found you could do it.

Negative self-talk is another example of how we can get in our own way. It gradually eats away at our self-esteem. Every time we tell ourselves we will try to do some exercise and then don't, we are breaking a promise we've made to ourselves.

If you said to a friend that you'll meet them at 10am and do Pilates with them, would you turn up? Would you keep that promise? I'd like to guess that unless there was a genuine emergency, you would keep your word, because that's good manners.

What if the person you had an appointment with at 10am to do Pilates with was you? Would you turn up? If you said 'No', that's fine. I broke my promises to myself hundreds of times a few years ago when it came to my exercise. I was not aware of how unkind I was being to myself and didn't know any different. I didn't value myself. Once you have this awareness, then it's your choice.

If you said 'Yes', great. You are honouring your promise to yourself.

When you make that promise and follow through, it boosts your self-esteem and restores your self-integrity. You feel good.

Get Thinking

1. What things do you say to yourself about your exercise?

List them here:

Now you have brought awareness to your self-talk, I want you to write a reframe for it.

For example, "I can't do this" could become "I can't do this yet" or even better, eliminating the word 'can't' you could say, "I am getting better at this all the time".

"I'm going to try to do some exercise today" could become, "I am going to move and be active today".

"I should do Pilates today" could become, "I am choosing to do Pilates today" or "I get to do Pilates today".

2. Write your reframes here:

Try them on, say them out loud to yourself and start using them in your language. Make sure they are positive, encouraging and kind. Be kind with what you say to yourself.

Time is an illusion

"Time is a puzzle, but understand how your beliefs about time shape your life and you can change the picture.'

Blyth (2018 p69)

Have you ever noticed how time shows up differently depending on what you are doing?

Have you ever tried to hold a plank position (facing the floor and supporting yourself on your forearms and toes) for 1 minute? It can feel like hours, as time seems to slow down.

Watch a good film for 2 hours though and the time just flies by.

My biggest obstacle to doing exercise when my children were little was my relationship with time.

In March 2019, I knew I wanted to help all those women that were not able to get to my community classes because of work or childcare and so had decided to offer Pilates online. I had no idea where to start but I invested in a training course to help me.

The first module of this course was all about my identity as an entrepreneur, and the business mentor asked me the same question I am going to ask you in a moment.

"What is your story around time? How do you see time?"

I wrote down in my workbook, because I'm that sort of person who likes to write everything down:

"I just haven't got enough time" or "I'm too busy".

He then said, "OK, what are you avoiding or not being responsible for by saying this?"

My answer was: "What do you mean?" (it was a recorded video, so I think I even said this out loud and with some defiance), "I'm not avoiding any responsibility, I do everything for everyone!"

So, before I continue with my story:

Get Thinking

What is your story around time? What do you say about time?

How does this make you feel when you say these things?

What are you avoiding or not being responsible for by saying this?

You might have said something similar to what I had said, or you may already be aware of what I was struggling to admit to myself.

If you feel like I felt, ask yourself the question again:

What are you avoiding or not being responsible for by saying this?

When I had the realisation of what I was avoiding taking responsibility for, it shifted my mindset massively and ultimately has led me to where I am now.

I was avoiding taking responsibility for myself. That really hit me but was the lesson I needed in order to grow and be a better version of myself.

Again, the words we use around time are not always helpful. We talk about how we 'spend' our time. The word 'spend' suggests that we don't get it back. If we think of 'investing' our time in something of value, then we will reap the rewards in the short and the more distant future.

All you need to do is change your story around time. Stop chasing it, stop rushing, and make time your friend. ***Enjoy time.***

Get Thinking

Catch yourself every time you say something that about no time, being busy, spending time.

Reframe it with: I have enough time to do everything I want to do, or I choose to do Pilates, or I am investing my time in me. Write down a few phrases you can use to reframe your story around time.

Say your new phrases out loud a few times. How do they make you feel?

Practise, practise, practise. It took me a long time to break the habit of saying I was busy. Soon after I'd completed this module in my business programme, I made a commitment to myself and told my husband, so he could help me, to banish my old-time stories and sayings. I decided that I would never say, "I haven't got enough time" or that "I am too busy" ever again. And I'm pleased to say, 3 years later, I have a positive and productive relationship with time and I always have plenty of time.

> *"Those who think they have no time
> to exercise, will sooner or later
> have to find time for illness.'*
>
> Edward Stanley, English clergyman 1779-1849

Re-energise

Another big obstacle that I have experienced, and I know other women have too, is not having enough energy to exercise.

Get Moving

Let's re-energise.

Stand up, sweep your arms up and take in a deep breath, then exhale as you lower your arms. Repeat three times. Then repeat again and as you exhale and your arms come down, take your chin to your chest and bend down, but do this by rolling down through your spine, one vertebra at a time. You can keep your legs bent or straight, whichever works best for you.

As you reach the floor, walk your hands forward until you are making an upside down 'V' shape with your body. Keep your hips high, with your head hanging between your arms, and your hands and feet grounded.

Take three deep breaths here, and each time you exhale, allow your chest to relax towards the ground and your spine to lengthen.

Walk your hands back in, legs bent or straight, and slowly, slowly, roll back up, one vertebra at a time, finishing with your head balancing on top of your tall spine.

Feel free to repeat this again if you want to.

Did you do it? Do you feel refreshed and energised?

A mum said to me a few years ago that when she feels like she's got the energy to exercise, she runs out of time to do it and then when she *does* have time, she feels too tired.

What she was doing was swapping one obstacle for another, and the outcome was that she could never do any exercise.

We can feel tired for many reasons other than a poor night's sleep. Making decisions, learning, meeting new people, multitasking, distractions, interruptions, these all require additional energy. I will talk more about some of these things in the next chapter, because if we can eliminate or reduce these things, we will feel less mentally exhausted.

When we are mentally exhausted, we have less motivation and are more likely to make decisions that give us instant gratification, such as collapsing on the sofa with a glass of wine.

When we are mentally energised, we are more likely to make decisions that benefit us now and in the long term, making us more likely to stick with our plans to exercise.

Saying we are just too tired to exercise is backwards thinking.

Let's just flip this on its head for the moment. When you have done a Pilates class, how do you feel? Refreshed? Energised? Positive? Ready to take on the world again?

That's how I feel after Pilates, and I know this is how all my clients over the years have felt.

It's not that you haven't got enough energy to exercise, it is that you need to get moving to re-energise.

Where's your motivation?

Do you feel as if you haven't got the motivation to exercise? Maybe you've told yourself this.

There are two types of motivation: **intrinsic** and **extrinsic**. Intrinsic motivation comes from within and involves doing something because it is personally rewarding. Being intrinsically motivated is typically a more effective method for long-term success. Extrinsic motivation comes from external rewards or punishment, which can be helpful but may lose effectiveness over time.

"The ultimate form of intrinsic motivation is when a habit becomes part of your identity. It's one thing to say I'm the type of person who <u>wants</u> this. It's something very different to say I'm the type of person who <u>is</u> this".

Clear (2018 p33)

So, to find your motivation you need to look inside you.

Get Thinking

I want you to write down here: Why do you want to exercise and move?

Great! But now dig deeper! Keep asking why to your answer above.

E.g., I want to exercise so I can go on a skiing holiday next year.

OK, why?

Well, because I want to enjoy the holiday and don't want to injure myself.

OK, why?

Because I want to join in with my family, and if I'm injured, I can't do that.

OK, why?

Because I want to create those memories with my family, be active and feel strong and capable.

OK, why?

You get the picture. I want you to keep asking yourself why, until you reach an answer that really connects with your emotionally, one you can really feel in your heart.

That is your intrinsic motivation.

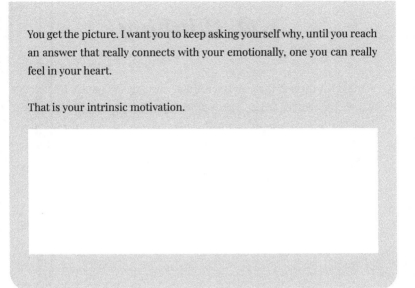

Every time you start to talk yourself out of being physically active, come back here and remind yourself WHY you are doing it.

Summary

By reflecting on your identity, values and beliefs you have increased your awareness of who you have been and how you have got in your own way. So, let's imagine who you want to be, what you say to yourself and what's important to you.

Get Thinking

Take a moment to imagine and then write down who you want to be. Write it in the present tense. E.g., I am a fit, strong, active woman who chooses to do Pilates. I enjoy moving my body, I have enough time and energy to do what is important to me, I am responsible for my health and fitness, I love looking after myself and I am just as important as everyone else.

Write it down and stick it up where you can see it.

Say this to yourself every day, visualise what your life would look like by being this person and *be* this person.

'*Becoming the best version of yourself requires you to continuously edit your beliefs, and to upgrade and expand your identity*'.

Clear (2018 p36)

Chapter 5

To Be or not to Be

*Y*ou have now decided 'who' you want to be. This is then reflected in everything you do – your habits. This is the second element of the Triangle of Strength.

Let me give you an example.

A person's identify might be that they are a smoker. What habits does a smoker have? Well, they buy cigarettes and smoke. If a person is not a smoker, then they do not have the habit of buying cigarettes or smoking them.

Every little thing you do every day, such as your habits, accumulate over time, whether they are good or bad. You can choose what these little things are, and when you choose how to be based on what is important to you, you are living in alignment with your values and living on purpose.

In this chapter I am going to talk about the characteristics of being that I have come across and seen in myself and in other women which allow us to develop powerful habits, powerful ways of being that empower us on our journey to become our best self for ourselves and for others.

I'll share with you the same strategies that I, and the women I've helped, have used successfully. Some may be more relevant to you than others depending on your current habits and way of being.

Be patient

Have you ever made a New Year's resolution? Most of us have at some point in our lives.

Did you keep your resolution past February?! No, me neither!

And that's because making a New Year's resolution is flawed. We make too many resolutions that are unrealistic, and without putting fundamental steps in place to help us achieve them, we are disappointed and give up when 4 weeks later we don't see any changes or progress. James Clear in his book *Atomic Habits* explains that this is because we focus on the goal rather than the systems we need to put in place to achieve them.

James Clear also states that it takes an average of 66 days to build a new habit. That's 2 months, and it may take some of us longer depending on the habit and how established old habits were.

If you want to make a new fitness-related habit, then it's important to remember that not only does building the habit take time but seeing the results does too.

Any improvement in strength, flexibility or change in your physical body takes time. Remember that if you see an advert on social media that claims you can get a 6-pack in 21 days or a toned bootie in a week or a bikini body in 14 days, this is a hook and is unrealistic for most of us. Now, yes it may be possible – I've never tried, but based on my own experience and knowledge for most of us who cannot spend every waking hour in the gym or have a chef to plan our meals or are prepared to live off a restricted diet or can solely commit to this one goal, these claims are misleading, and I could imagine lead to injury, malnutrition or frustration.

Changing your physical body safely and sustainably takes time.

> *'Patience and persistence are vital qualities*
> *in the ultimate successful accomplishment*
> *of any worthwhile endeavour'.*
>
> Pilates (1945, p11)

Often, we think of making progress as a linear, diagonal upward path, but in reality, the line of progress may plateau or even drop slightly whilst the effects of your daily small habits gain momentum and accumulate.

Progress is still progress though, however small.

> *"The process of building habits is*
> *actually the process of becoming*
> *yourself. This is a gradual evolution'.*
>
> Clear (2018 p37)

Ever done a workout and felt really good? You've been able to do more repetitions of a particular exercise, or a harder level and the movement feels smoother and more controlled but then the next time you do it, it feels like you've gone backwards – you can't do the same number of repetitions or the harder level and you are wobbling all over the place.

This is not because you've got worse. It doesn't mean anything – it's one workout, a snapshot in time. Think of your progress by looking at the big picture.

All your small habits build up over time:

- Standing up from your desk every 30 minutes will help relieve your backache.
- Stretching your hamstrings for 5 minutes every day will help you to touch your toes by the end of the year.

- Doing 10 push-ups every day will maintain your upper body strength so you can garden without aching.
- Engaging your core, dropping your shoulders and bringing your ears in line with your shoulders every 20 minutes will result in a better standing posture a year later.
- Telling yourself you are a fit, strong and healthy woman every morning will become your default identity after 12 months.

The magic is in the mundane.

Be organised

I love lists! I love planning and I am ultra-organised! This is part of my identity. It helps me to juggle a family of 5 and a dog, everyone's different activities, even if some weekends it is a bit of a military operation (and of course this way of living is my choice).

As a child I always remember my mum saying, "Gila – stop organising the game and just play." But for me the best bit was organising it.

I'll give you an example of my organisational skills from a young age, but this on its own was not enough to hold me accountable to do any exercise.

Now, have you ever heard of 'The Bobble Club'?

If you were to ask my brothers and sister what their most memorable moment of our childhoods was, they would say 'The Bobble Club'. Now, I am the eldest of 4, I have two younger brothers and a younger sister. I was aware when I was about 11 or 12 that my mum and dad never had any time to themselves, so I started a club to entertain my siblings and give my mum and dad time off!

I was the Head of course. My eldest brother was Deputy Head, my next youngest brother was Deputy, Deputy Head and yes, you've guessed it, my little sister was Deputy, Deputy, Deputy Head.

Joining fee = 50p (if you haven't got it, ask Mum)

Membership – includes a badge with your role on and a weekly newsletter with puzzles and games. (If you lost your badge, and my younger brother did, you had to pay 50p for a new one!).

Venue – my bedroom, every Sunday at 2pm.

Club activities – bring a plastic ruler and bang on my bedroom floor to try to make a hole so a fireman's pole can be fitted from my bedroom down to the garage below!

In case you are wondering – I never did get a fireman's pole from my bedroom down to the garage – you won't be surprised to know that our efforts were in vain.

Clearly, I was not meant to go into structural engineering – but I was already refining my skills in organising and planning. (Little did I know that The Bobble Club was my first membership and that 30 years later I'd be running a Pilates membership).

As a primary school teacher my organisational skills enable me to plan for different abilities, learners, and subjects. I've organised gym and dance displays, conferences and many school sports acrobatics competitions. So, with all that experience, you'd think I'd be able to plan in my own exercise to my schedule.

But here's what I've learned.

A plan that looks like this:

'I'll do my exercise at some point today', doesn't work.

A plan that says, 'I'll aim to do it before lunch', doesn't work.

What you think your plan looks like

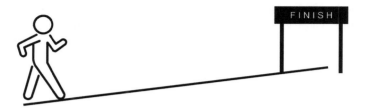

What your plan actually looks like

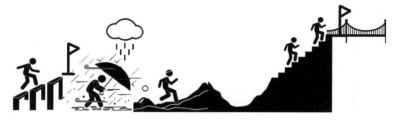

Creating your Movement Accountability Statement

You can be great at planning and organising but the bit I missed for a long time was that once I'd made a plan, I had to actually follow through on it. My plan wasn't specific, and I didn't prioritise my exercise. It was always at the end of my 'To Do' list and hence always got missed off. This was also down to me not having a positive mindset at the time.

Your plan needs to be a Movement Accountability Statement, which is written down, and in doing so you make a silent pact with yourself. My clients and I use this approach and it's a highly successful way to help women to get into the habit of making time to move and exercise.

There are four essential ingredients: The What, the When, the Where and the Who.

What

What type of movement are you going to do? E.g., Bitesize Pilates Core Workout.

As James Clear states in his book *Atomic Habits*, it is a craving that will lead to action. You will find it an easier habit to build if you have a desire to do it. So, choose an activity that you enjoy and want to do.

When

When are you going to do it? E.g., Monday morning at 6.30am.

This might be different each day or the same, it doesn't matter. I have some members who are like clockwork and at 6.30am every morning they check in with me and tell me they've done their Pilates session. Other members, it varies each day.

You can attach your movement session to something else in your routine which has to happen, to help you to stick with it. For example, if your toddler has some planned downtime, a snack and watches their favourite programme at the same time each day, that could be an opportunity for you to get moving.

Where

Where are you going to do it? I call this your Success Space.

As a teacher, the staffroom table would nearly always have a box of assorted chocolates on the table. I'd walk in and eat a few, even though the thought of eating chocolate had not entered my head previously. James Clear in his book *Atomic Habits* explains various research that has been conducted to demonstrate how visual humans are and how this affects our behaviour. This is often used to manipulate how we shop, with more expensive products being placed at eye level and cheaper products on the bottom shelf.

We can design our environment positively to help us create good habits such as doing Pilates. Create a space where you want to move and make it easy and accessible. If your space is dominated by your TV and you have to get your mat out of the boot of the car, but the remote is right there in front of you, it will be easier to choose to just sit down and watch television.

Creating your Success Space

1. Have your clothes out ready, have your mat in view, with your resistance band or other small equipment you may want in an attractive basket or on a shelf. Add a plant, a different light or an inspirational picture.
2. Remove distractions such as piles of washing or toys.
3. Turn off notifications or move away from your computer.
4. Visualise yourself enjoying moving and indulging in yourself in this space, feeling calm and strong.
5. Keep this book where you can see it, so it is a reminder to hold yourself accountable.

One of my clients was working from home, looking at the computer screen and having meetings on Zoom all day, and then was looking at the same screen, standing in the same space to follow her online Bitesize Pilates. She found the Pilates wasn't helping her switch off and clear her mind like she knew it could from her own previous experience of doing Pilates at my community class. She was no longer able to get to the community class but wanted to continue her Pilates to give her a break from work.

Together we worked on her taking a 'commute' from her work in one room of her house to a different room in her house which was for her Pilates class. She was experienced at doing Pilates and could just listen to my instructions. There were no distractions from work, email notifications or paperwork. The room had more natural light and had her mat waiting ready. She added a plant or two. Now she had a different environment to do her Pilates in and although nothing else had changed, she was able to 'leave' work and 'go' to Pilates, and this physical shift in space allowed her to shift her brain from 'work mode' to 'me time'. She then regained all the mental benefits from Pilates that she wanted.

Who

Being accountable to someone helps you to stay on track and establish new habits. I encourage all my clients to have an accountability partner, and for some clients, that is me! They check in with me each day to tell me they've done a Pilates session. This helps them to stick with the promises they've made to themselves because they know I'll be asking them how they've got on when we have a progress call, which I do every 90 days.

Find yourself an accountability partner. Someone who is:

a. Trustworthy
b. Non judgmental
c. Honest
d. Encouraging
e. Challenging
f. Gives constructive feedback
g. Emotionally resilient
h. Knows you can do it
i. Gives unconditional support
j. Gives you a break

Then ask them and get their agreement.

Get Thinking

Write down your Movement Accountability Statement

What... (something you want to do)

When.... (be specific)

Where... (create your Success Space)

Who... (name of accountability partner)

However, we all know life likes to throw us a curveball and so we need to be ready with a Plan B and possibly a Plan C too!

I could list you at least 27 excuses that I've heard over the years, as to why women haven't been able to do their Pilates (some are my own!). Everything from, 'It's too dark and cold' to 'I had to clean the kitchen', to 'I had to work'.

Instead of allowing these obstacles to block our way, we just need to re-prioritise in our mind the importance of moving. A highly successful approach that I use with my clients and myself is to have accountability. Accountability with yourself by having a Plan A and Plan B, or accountability from a teacher, or accountability by having both: a plan and a teacher.

Find a way that works for you to get past your obstacles, jump over them, go round them, knock them flat but don't let them stop you moving.

Get Thinking

Write your Plan B for as many obstacles you can think of that may stop you doing any exercise/movement, using the sentence template: 'If... then'.

For example:

If my child is poorly, then I will do my Pilates once my partner is home to look after them.

Or

If I need to work late Friday evening, then I will do my Pilates session on Saturday morning.

Another key point that has really helped me is to write down my plan the night before so that the next day the decision has already been made. Done! If you take just 5 minutes planning the next day the night before, it will save you an hour of your precious time making that decision, procrastinating and ruminating on it during the following day.

That's worth doing, isn't it?

Be clear

You know your values. You have a plan. Now you can prioritise your actions and ensure they align with your values.

'Do first things first and second things not at all.'

Tracy (2017, p28)

Avoid my mistake. I would plan my exercise in but not as a priority. My family and my work would always take precedent and my exercise 'time slot' would get squeezed. I would find myself just tying up some loose ends, emails and messages that had just come through and then aim to start my exercise a few minutes later than planned. But a few minutes would turn into 10, then 15 and then my exercise time would become almost non-existent. So, I'd try to squeeze it in, but that's not a mindset that helps you feel good about it. The only thing I should be squeezing are my glutes not my time!

If you feel rushed, you don't fully focus, you don't concentrate on what you are doing whilst moving, you're not 'in the zone'. This is just as bad as planning it and not doing it at all. By squeezing it in I was still not valuing myself. I would have been better just deciding not to do it and be happy with that choice.

If this was an appointment with someone else, would you turn up 15 minutes late and rush the session, not really giving it your full attention? I would feel terrible doing that to any of my clients, and, in any work (or indeed social) situation, if someone did that to you, how would you feel? Why do this to yourself? What does it tell you about what you think of yourself?

For me, I realised that although I was planning in my exercise and my approach was loads better than previously, I was still not truly aligning my actions with my values and so still left feeling rubbish about myself. When your actions don't align with your values, you have that dissatisfied, frustrated, guilty feeling because you haven't done what you wanted to do or what you said you would do.

'Make up your mind that you will perform your Contrology [Pilates] exercise ten minutes without fail. Amazingly enough, once you travel on this Contrology 'Road to Health' you will subconsciously lengthen your trip on it from 10 to 20 or more minutes before you realise it.'

Pilates (1945, p11)

Get Thinking

When planning, prioritise your daily tasks so they align with your values.

Write down your daily tasks.

Go back to your values from the last chapter.

Add 1-5 (1 = highest value) next to each one and check that what you are doing aligns with your values. Do your actions match your values?

By doing this exercise you can be clear that you are living on purpose and are at peace with your choices because you're doing what's important to you.

Be committed

I touched on this at the start of the book, and if you're still here reading this, that should tell you that already you are being committed.

When we are 100% committed, we've made the decision to do something, no matter what. Having made this decision makes it easier for us to follow through.

How many times have you had a conversation with yourself about whether you should do your exercise or not? My biggest debate was always exercise or work. It sounded like this:

Gila (inner voice): Shall I go to my exercise class tonight?

Gila Monster (self-sabotaging voice): If you stay home, you could finish answering your emails and you really should do that.

Gila: But I could do that tomorrow and I have paid for the class.

Gila Monster: But people will be waiting for a reply and if you don't reply tonight, they might go elsewhere, and you'll lose business.

Gila: But I'll feel better when I've done my exercise and a few more hours to reply won't make any difference – no-one will check emails tonight.

This sort of conversation is mentally exhausting and just leaves you feeling drained and too tired to make any decision.

You'll recognise this feeling if you've ever taken on some home renovation. You need to decide where you want plug switches, what type of shelves you need, what shade of paint, what floor tiles and what type of lighting... too many decisions and you become a bit punch drunk, because it takes energy to make decisions.

However, now you know your values, making decisions is easier, and when your decisions align with your values, you will feel good about them. When making decisions it will also help to know your boundaries and protect them.

If you say 'Yes' to one thing, you are saying 'No' to something else.

Too often I would say 'Yes' to help someone else, which resulted in me then not having time to exercise.

I love making cakes and have always made cakes for my children for their birthdays. A few years ago, I posted some of the cakes I'd made on Facebook and all of a sudden, I started getting requests to make cakes.

Often, I'd get a request two days before the cake was needed and I'd say 'Yes' because I wanted to help, and I'll admit I was flattered to be asked. I'd end up working non-stop and into the night to finish the cake, aiming for perfection. My neck, shoulders and back would ache – I really would have benefitted from doing Pilates but it was the first thing to go as I'd committed my time to making cakes.

By saying 'Yes' to make a cake at short notice for friends, I was saying 'No' to my time for exercise.

If at that time, I had been clear about what was important to me and had stopped to reflect on my values, then saying no would have been easy. I could have replied, "No, but I can do it for next week". This would have allowed me to plan my time better and have more realistic deadlines, or I could have just said 'No' and I'm sure they would have found someone else.

Saying no is powerful and when you have the courage and confidence to say it, a massive weight lifts from your shoulders.

I'd like you to do this the next time someone asks you to do something. Stop giving an immediate, automatic answer and instead, perhaps get back to them later with your answer once you have had time to decide if it aligns with your values. This gives you the time to weigh up more clearly, if you say yes what will have to go?

If it's your physical activity that will have to go, how will that make you feel?

If you said 'No', what would happen? How would that make you feel?

Unless you protect your boundaries and say no, and choose how to spend your time, others will soon spend it for you.

Get Thinking

List the things you do at the moment, or often agree to do, that are stealing your time from being physically active:

Look through your list and write the word 'NO' in big capital letters next to those things that you are going to say 'NO' to and free up some time for the things you WANT to say 'Yes' to.

List down what things you say 'YES' to: These will align with your values you identified in Chapter 4.

Stephen Covey, in his book *7 Habits of Highly Effective People,* explores the distinction between important tasks and urgent tasks. This is another way to help you focus on the things in your life that will help you to live a happy and fulfilling life.

Even when we know what our highest values are, our attention and time can easily be diverted by urgent things that demand our attention, for example a phone ringing. The phone call may or may not be important.

Some distractions are neither urgent or important and may just be pleasurable or easy e.g., scrolling through social media, watching re-runs of *Friends*, yet we will still find ourselves spending our time on them.

Our health is of fundamental importance but it does not demand our immediate attention. It is only when your back gives way and starts causing pain that it then becomes urgent and important. We then take notice and do something about it. Once the pain, the symptom, subsides, many of us then stop exercising and moving, forgetting the urgency and not addressing the cause of the problem (which was likely to have been a lack of strength and mobility). We stop prioritising our health and fitness until the next time our back causes us pain. Even though our health can gradually decline through physical inactivity, many of us will take the risk that we will be OK. This is because we don't have a strong enough inclination to exercise even though we understand it is important.

I believe we need to harness our understandable bias towards instant gratification and the attraction of the path of least resistance by moving in a way that is simple, easy and enjoyable. Don't fight it – work with it! We will then crave that 'feel good feeling' and want to move more, move better and move for longer.

Get Thinking

1. Write a list of the types of things that are important to you.

2. Which of these are urgent and which are not urgent?

3. Write a list of the types of things that are not important to you.

4. Which of these are urgent or not urgent?

5. Where do you place most of your attention and time?

If your list contains many urgent but non-important items, then, like me a few years ago, this is what is keeping you busy but still making you feel like you are not achieving anything you want to.

If most of your attention is on non-important and non-urgent things, why? What reward are you getting from doing these things?

Ideally, we want to spend most of our time on the things that are important to us, but there may be some urgent things along the way that demand our attention. It's then up to you how much attention you give them.

> *'Not only is health a normal condition, but it is a duty not only to attain it, but to maintain it.'*
>
> Pilates (1934, p12)

Be free

Being in control is a double-edged sword. I like to be in control and feel in control; however, I have also had to learn to let go of control.

My belief was that being in control meant I had to do everything, whether this was in my family, my job, my business, in every aspect of my life – except of course when it came down to looking after myself. During those years when my children were very little the one thing I wasn't in control of was my fitness.

I felt I was the only one who could look after my children, the only one who could look after my house, teach my class, and do my job.

When I was a teacher, I would always dread it when I had to go on a course for the day and had to leave cover for a supply teacher. I believed that no one would be able to teach my class and look after them as well as I could, and I'd worry that the next day there would be loads of issues I'd have to deal with.

And you know what? The next day the children were fine, their education hadn't been affected and 9 times out of 10 there were no pieces to put back together. I was younger then and didn't see how this need for control was not helping me. It took me a long time to learn the lesson of letting go.

I would decide to do my exercise in the evening when the children were in bed. I'd help get them washed, teeth brushed, into pyjamas, bedtimes stories read – one each, tuck them in and say goodnight. I'd collect the washing and start downstairs. Have you ever noticed the knack children have of shouting for you just as you are about halfway down the stairs? "Mummy!"

Then the delaying tactics would start...

"Can I have a drink please?"

"I need a hot water bottle."

"I don't want to go to school tomorrow."

"Can I show you something?"

Once all these were sorted, I'd finally get downstairs and I'd get my mat out, take a deep breath and even then, one of my children would appear at the door. "Mummy... I can't find..." (whatever object was vital to find immediately).

You get the idea, and I'm sure you've experienced bedtimes like these if you have children. Before I knew it, my patience was being tested, I'd look at the clock, 10 minutes of the time I'd allocated had gone and I'd start to feel cross and a voice in my head would say, 'This isn't fair, I'm just trying to do some exercise for me, is this too much to ask?'

What wasn't fair was expecting my family to respect this time for me, when 1) I didn't respect it for myself and 2) I hadn't communicated with them what I was trying to do.

My need to be in control had taught my children that they didn't need to think for themselves and need not respect my time, because until that point, I hadn't respected my time either.

As soon as I explained my intentions and that I'd like their help with what I was trying to do, protecting my boundaries and being purposeful with my time was clearer for me and my family.

It took some practice and I'm not saying it's perfect now but by letting go of control I have gained more control over how I want to live.

Be trusting

This follows on, as it uses the same thought process as that used to gain more control. To let go of the limiting aspects of control it is easier if you trust others and trust yourself.

Trust people to do things for themselves, and trust others to do things to help you.

There is simply not enough time to do everything so the magic here is to delegate. Delegate the things you don't like doing or that someone else can do at least 80% as well as you can, if not better. Remember, perfection doesn't exist.

This will give you back the time to do all the things that only you can do and that you do best.

You are the only one that can do your push-ups, and we'll explore this more in the next chapter.

Trust yourself to say no. Trust that you know what you want – which you do now – by reading this book.

Trust yourself.

Trust others.

Get Moving

Active rest is just as important as purposeful movement.

Take a moment and give your brain a rest by taking some time to focus on your breathing.

Stop. Sit, stand or lay down. Take a deep breath in and then out.

Breathe in, filling the lungs with fresh oxygen and then exhale, allowing every last drop of air to escape, taking with it anything you no longer need.

Do this cycle three more times. I like to close my eyes too and feel the movement of my ribcage rising and falling.

Feel better?

Be consistent

Consistency is key.

Being consistent is about repeating the same thing over and over again, improving a little bit each time.

In July 2019, I created a magical moment by performing an aerial silks routine with my daughter, who was 6 at the time.

She chose the music, 'Never Enough' from *The Greatest Showman*. It's a moment I will never forget and had the audience in tears!

I think the only reason I didn't cry during the performance was because I was concentrating on the routine and on making sure my daughter was OK.

I hadn't performed in front of an audience for a long time, over 10 years in fact, and both my daughter and I were, as you'd expect, feeling nervous. It doesn't matter how many times I've performed before, I still get nervous.

It had been about 6 months earlier that we had decided to do a silks routine together. In that time, we practised, we repeated the same moves, the same routine, over and over again. We tweaked the timing, we practised in costumes, our teacher gave us feedback about whether we should look towards each other or to the audience at different points, if our arms were in the same alignment or if a position was better with a straight leg or bent.

Every week we practised together at the studio, together at home off the silks and I practised on my own every week too.

We needed to practise every week at least, to improve the routine and moves, retain and improve our strength and stamina to perform it, make it look effortless, to be able to remember the routine and increase our confidence.

If we had only managed a few ad hoc practices here and there in the months leading up to the show our performance would not have been as polished, confident or as enjoyable as it was. The same as you don't win an Olympic gold medal by rocking up to training two weeks before.

Being consistent and regular, practising the same moves over and over again and improving it each time, resulted in an amazing performance.

To get better at anything, you need to practise, and if you are consistent, you will get the results you are after quicker, as long as you are focused on the right things.

To be consistent, as a busy woman, you need to find a way to incorporate movement into your lifestyle that is easy. If you can do it easily, you will be able to remain consistent, and if you are consistent, you'll see and feel your progress, notice the physical and mental difference and enjoy being physically active.

Being consistent though, does not mean you have to be consistent 100% of the time or that any time you miss a session or don't do Pilates means you've failed. Absolutely not. Maybe this is true if you are training as a top athlete and your aim is to win at a world championship. Remember, perfection doesn't exist and there is more to life than exercising. For me, Pilates gives me the physical strength and mental clarity to be able to enjoy all the other things I want to do in life whilst looking after myself.

To be a fit, strong and active woman doesn't mean that your whole life has to revolve around exercise, unless of course you want it to.

Michael Matthews explains in his *Little Black Book of Workout Motivation* that you need to be consistent at least 80% of the time.

Have you ever seen fit, slim people out at a restaurant and wonder how they can eat such a big meal and have dessert and not get fat? That's because that meal is a one-off, not a daily habit. They enjoy the big meal and pudding and then the next day they are eating healthy food and sensible portion sizes again.

If 80 days out of 100, you are active, move, stretch, do some strength training, go for a walk, eat nutritious meals, what will be the outcome?

Correct – you'll be fitter, stronger, feel better physically and mentally, and you'll be healthier. You will BE an active, strong, healthy woman. This will become your identity. You are not obsessed with getting a 6-pack, you are just being the type of person who doesn't miss a session. Keeping track of your sessions also enables you to focus on remaining consistent and it is rewarding to cross off a session each time you do it. (Clear (2018)) My members have a monthly programme and use a progress tracker that helps them do just that, remain consistent. It is a visual reminder.

Here's another example of how small daily habits add up to huge rewards. Darren Hardy calls it, in his book of the same name: The Compound Effect.

Would you rather have £3million pounds now or 1p today which doubles every day for 31 days?

Well, £3million right now sounds pretty good, right? Think about what you could do with that money!

However, if you do the maths and can remain consistent, over the long term the benefits far outweigh the immediate gratification. 1p doubled every day for 31 days gives you £10.7 million! And this is the same with your health: do you go for the quick fix or be patient and wait for the long-term rewards – but you only get those long-term rewards if you are consistent?

When it comes to your health and fitness, quick fixes can be as simple as taking painkillers. If you suffer from backache from long periods of inactivity and weak core strength, painkillers are an option. However, I would argue that this route does not address the cause of the problem. The tablets do not strengthen your core muscles or help to mobilise your spine.

There is no magic pill!

Yet, moving your body does release endorphins, natural 'feel good' chemicals that relieve pain, stress and make you feel good! It has been said that movement is medicine.

I don't believe there are any quick fixes when it comes to building strength and improving flexibility. Remaining consistent with moving daily will have a positive ripple effect on the rest of your life.

Be calm

My alarm clock rings, waking me up with a start, still feeling tired and like I've been run over by a bus. Our puppy has decided that 4.30am is the best time to get up and chase squirrels or leaves blowing in the wind, and he doesn't want to settle down. So, I have not had a very restful night's sleep and had just about managed to doze back off when the alarm clock sounds at 6am.

I go downstairs to get breakfast and the milk has gone off, my youngest son starts whining that he doesn't want to go to school and that his slippers are uncomfortable, which is made no better by collapsing on the kitchen floor. My other two children start arguing because one of them has looked at the other in a certain way.

My husband comes in from taking the dog for a walk in the pouring rain and now there is a new pile of washing and a wet, muddy dog running around the dining room table.

My eldest then says he has some homework to do that he has forgotten to do and needs help with.

After finally sorting breakfast, listening to reading, helping with homework, mopping up after a spilt drink and cuddling my daughter because she'd banged her head on the fridge door, because I'd left it open to get some fresh milk out, everyone is dressed and ready for the day.

My youngest cries all the way as we walk to school, because his socks are now uncomfortable.

I walk back to the car and take a deep breath. What a morning... and it's not even 9.00am. Have you ever had a morning, a day, a week like that?

The rest of my day continues with email and social media notifications, business meetings, messages from my children's schools, washing to do so PE kit is clean for the next day, cooking, cleaning, children's activities, Pilates (of course!) and so on, until 9pm, I take the dog out again for an evening walk round the block and shower and bed.

What I've described is life! Even when everything is good, life can feel overwhelming. If you let it.

Several years ago, I quite often felt overwhelmed and mentally drained by the end of the day.

The world we live in can feel chaotic, fast, busy, unfair and unhappy. This external world is out of our control. The only things we can control are the thoughts we choose to focus on and how we feel.

When I became aware of this, I realised I could choose to feel overwhelmed by life or I could embrace it, because it was a life I had created.

When I had said to myself that I should really try and do some exercise today and then didn't for all the reasons I've already explored with you, it was because I was choosing to feel overwhelmed with everything I had chosen to do, overwhelmed with looking after everyone else, overwhelmed with making decisions, overwhelmed trying to meet unspoken expectations, and this choice was leaving me mentally drained.

I've now learnt that I can choose my internal world, my feelings, and choose not to be overwhelmed. Just knowing this has made life so much lighter.

When you are feeling overwhelmed, these things might help you, as they help me:

1. Tell yourself everything will work out just as it should. Life is happening for you.
2. Just stop and breathe. Step back from the doing, being busy. Decide you are not going to feel overwhelmed.
3. Take 20 minutes to do a short Pilates session and this has always helped me quiet my mind.
4. Be grateful. Take a moment to think about what you have got. Would you want it any other way?

Get Moving

Take a break from reading this book and go get moving. Go for a walk, stretch, walk up and down stairs, take the stairs instead of the lift, fidget, stand on one leg whilst brushing your teeth. Do whatever you want but just get moving.

Be your best self

Being our best self takes practice.

Get Thinking

Look back at your description at the end of Chapter 4.

What will you change in order to be this way?

What little habits do you need to do every day to be your best self?

What help do you need and who from?

What's stopping you being your best self now?

What will you change first, what's the one thing?

What would your ripple effect be if you were being your best self?

Chapter 6

You're the only one who can do your push ups

*F*or you to build strength, improve your flexibility and feel good about yourself, you have to move your own body. Moving is one of a few things (along with sleeping, going to the toilet and eating) that you and only you can do. These are things that you can't delegate. If you want to receive the benefits of movement the only way to do this is to do it yourself.

When I first started teaching Pilates, women would come to my classes and would say to me how good they felt afterwards and how much they enjoyed the class. But then I wouldn't see them for several weeks. They'd turn back up at class and say how much they'd missed it.

As a new Pilates teacher, I was confused and frustrated because why would they love coming to class and then not come? Why would they say they'd been recommended by their doctor to do Pilates to help with their backache and then not come? Why did they say they wanted a stronger core and then not come? I could only help these women if they came to class and actually did Pilates.

I now understand that it was not anything to do with my class, it was also not anything to do with childcare or having to work, certainly not in every case. It was to do with these women not placing enough importance on their health and fitness but allowing other things to take priority.

I wanted to help these women, because I too had been in a position when my health and fitness was not my priority either. When women join my Facebook group 'Bitesize Pilates for Busy Women', I ask the question: 'What's the one thing that stops you exercising?' The answer is nearly always 'time'.

The guaranteed way to improve your fitness, to get stronger and more flexible is by consistently and regularly moving. That's it! But if you can't be consistent and regular because you can't get to a class because you don't have time... well, you won't maintain, let alone improve, your fitness and health.

I believe that all the women of today need is a different approach to their health and fitness. When you have a busy schedule and you are juggling lots of different things, the simplest way to be consistent and sustain a regular routine is to move well and move little and often. Specific Pilates movements performed in bitesize chunks is flexible and can easily fit in with your lifestyle.

Research supports this approach as well. Schmidt et al. (2001) state that, 'Exercise accumulated in several short bouts has similar effects as one continuous bout'. O'Donovan et al, (2017) in a British study, concluded that there is more than one way to achieve your fitness goals and for time-poor people it is better to do little and often and fit it into their lifestyle.

This is how Bitesize Pilates evolved and it is this approach we use in CORE, my online Pilates membership. It is much easier to find 20 minutes of uninterrupted time and that time can be whenever it works for you. It doesn't need to be at the same time that a hall or an instructor is free.

Many of my founding members of CORE had done weekly Pilates classes with me face-to-face for many years prior to me opening the doors to CORE. Now, they wouldn't go back. They have told me how they are doing far more Pilates now than they ever did and feeling so much stronger than when they just did one hour once a week.

One client who is in her 60s told me how she, her husband and her son had been rebuilding a dry-stone wall. Her husband and her son were surprised that she could lift the stones and move them into place, but they were even more surprised when the next day she was the only one not complaining of her back aching and she was ready to go again. She does Bitesize Pilates consistently and regularly and I've taught her for over 14 years. She said how at the end of the day after mending this wall, she went and did her Pilates and that was what had not only given her the strength and mobility to be able to help with the wall in the first place but had also enabled her body to recover so quickly to continue working the next day.

Now, you might ask me, but why Pilates? Could I just not go for a run every day or a swim or go to the gym?

That's a good question. If you enjoy swimming, swim, if you enjoy running, run, do what you enjoy because then you are 90% of the way there into making it a consistent habit. (Clear (2018))

However, Pilates has some qualities that no other type of exercise can offer.

The power of Pilates

Joseph Pilates was a sickly child and suffered from asthma, rickets and rheumatic fever. He made it his mission to rebuild his body and reclaim his health. (www. pilatesfoundation.com/pilates/the-history-of-pilates)

Pilates 'builds a sturdy body and sound mind fitted to perform every daily task with ease and perfection as well as to provide tremendous reserve energy for sport, recreation and emergencies'. (Pilates (1945, p14))

When Joseph Pilates began to develop his system of movement, that he called 'Contrology', he worked mainly with ballet dancers and was influenced by ballet, gymnastics, boxing and tai chi.

Then Pilates became an exclusive type of fitness that only celebrities and world class athletes practiced, but today Pilates is available and accessible to more and more people. People like you and me. Osteopaths, chiropractors, doctors and other health care practitioners often prescribe Pilates to help improve spinal health and relieve back aches and pains. Pilates is performed by amateur and elite athletes and dancers. Pilates improves not only your physical health but your mental health too.

Have you ever been to a gym or fitness studio where you can cycle on an exercise bike or run on a treadmill and at the same time watch the news or catch up on the soaps on a big TV screen in front of you? You may have seen people exercising in this way and maybe have even done it yourself.

However, I'd like to ask you how much benefit you are getting from exercising like this. Are you thinking about your technique? Are you thinking about recruiting and working the right muscles? Are you thinking about your breathing and using it to help you? Are you focused on the quality of your movement and if you are working effectively and safely?

I expect the answer to each of those questions is 'No'. You are multitasking and therefore you are not able to do both tasks to the best of your ability. Part of your brain, the part that is controlling your movement, will likely be operating on autopilot as your brain is listening and taking in the new, visual information on the screen in front of you.

Pilates is a mindful movement

Joseph Pilates specifically designed his exercise system to engage the mind and the body. You concentrate on your breathing, the quality of your movement, you think about the muscles you are working and where your arms and legs are in space! It is this conscious conditioning of the body that makes Pilates the perfect 'exercise' for busy women.

When I worked as a primary school teacher, I would often end the day with a headache. This was probably due to not drinking enough water during the day, working with children, running clubs at lunchtimes and after school, aiming for perfection as a teacher and never giving myself a break.

I would arrive at Pilates to teach a class feeling so tired and drained that if I hadn't been teaching it, I would have just gone home and got in the bath and then probably eaten a whole load of chocolate in an attempt to make myself feel better.

Because I was running the class, I would take a deep breath and start teaching Pilates. Teaching Pilates was different from the school environment, because for a start everyone listened, they wanted to be there, and no one misbehaved! Even though I didn't physically do most of the class, for one hour I thought about and practised my breathing, I checked in on my posture, I moved my body and stretched.

And every single time, without exception, by the end of the class, my headache had gone. I felt refreshed and reenergised, and my mind felt clear. Everything that an hour before had felt like a heavy weight squashing me down, suddenly felt lighter. Everything felt alright again in the world.

Although Pilates is known for building core strength, improving posture, mobility and flexibility, for me it's not for these benefits alone. It is just as much, if not more, the clarity of mind, the energy and confidence I gain from doing Pilates.

In my 20 years of teaching Pilates, I have taught children through to women and men in their 70s and 80s. I've taught cyclists, dancers, climbers and runners. I've taught those who haven't been able to move their back for over 10 years and cannot bend down to tie their shoelaces, and I've taught those who are already physically very strong and mobile. I've taught people on mats, I've taught people on the stability ball and on the reformer (a piece of equipment Joseph Pilates designed); I've even taught some aerial Pilates!

I love Pilates because you start at your level, you work at your own pace and the only competition is with yourself – if you want it. Pilates can be adapted and modified so anyone can have the appropriate amount of challenge in order to make progress and can work safely and effectively.

So, anyone can do Pilates. You can do Pilates. Pilates is the most effective way for busy women to build strength, improve flexibility, increase circulation, improve balance and posture, relieve backache and feel good about yourself.

Pilates has stood the test of time

Pilates is not just for the time when you are doing a class – it's a lifestyle choice. It can be integrated and applied to every move you make during your day: walking around the supermarket, sat a desk, gardening or playing sports, because Pilates is about improving your functional movement capabilities.

A lot of fitness classes tend to work the body mostly in the sagittal plane, that is, forwards and backwards. However, our body, our muscles and joints are three-dimensional so we need to work in three planes of movement, forward and backward, side to side, and rotation, in order to move better. Pilates does all of this.

Pilates has stood the test of time because it works – it is not merely the latest fitness craze!

I believe it is also more relevant today than ever before because Pilates is about improving natural, functional movement and is the most effective way to be able to rebalance the effects of our sedentary and inactive lifestyle.

The other crucial advantage that Pilates has over other types of 'exercise' is that it is about quality not quantity. It's not about doing more. It's about doing it better. You can just do a few focused exercises every day and you will still get all the benefits, if not more, that you would from doing an hour's class once a week.

Pilates 'develops the body uniformly, corrects wrong postures, restores physical vitality, invigorates the mind and elevates the spirit.' (Pilates (1945, p9))

What's your goal when it comes to your fitness?

A lot of fitness influencers trade off how we want to look. They pose in bikinis and show their 6-pack or big bootie or whatever the latest trend is in how to look, and claim that if you follow their exercise routine you can get the same results. Well, I have not tried everyone's routine and cannot comment on their effectiveness but if your goal is solely to improve how you look in a bikini then Pilates may not be the right option for you.

My goal, through all my years of moving, has never been to improve how I look. I have done gymnastics and dancing, silks, walking, Pilates all because that's what I have enjoyed doing.

BUT the ripple effect of doing these activities *has* resulted in how I look. Pilates lengthens and tones muscles and many clients have said how their clothes fit better as a result. Their improved posture means they look and feel more confident. Pilates gives me and my clients the best of both worlds – *we can feel and look good, by doing something we enjoy.*

Get Moving

Kneel on the floor on your hands and knees.

Hands under your shoulders, knees under your hips.

Tuck your tailbone under, take your chin to your chest, look through your knees and round your back (this is a cat stretch).

Then reverse this movement, tilt your tailbone away and look up ahead of you, hollowing your spine (this is called a cow stretch!).

Repeat and do a few cat and cow stretches.

Now sit your tailbone back on your heels, keep your hands reaching forward on the mat and elbows lifted. Rest here for a couple of breaths.

Feel better?

What is Pilates?

'Pilates [Contrology] is the complete co-ordination of body, mind and spirit.'
Pilates (1945, p9)

The best way to know if you are going to enjoy it is to try it.

Give it a go. Not just one go, as you can't make an educated decision from just one session. Pick from the list below and do 5 or 6, then repeat them a few times so you get used to the movement. It will become easier each time.

Pilates for beginners

If you have never done Pilates before or have only done it a few times, that's OK.

> ### *'You don't have to be great to start, but you have to start to be great.'*
> Zig Ziglar

I'd recommend you start by watching my videos on the basic fundamentals of Pilates first and then do the session which introduces you to the basic levels of classic Pilates moves.

Learning anything new takes time, perseverance and practice.

> ### *'PATIENCE and PERSISTENCE are vital qualities in the ultimate successful accomplishment of any worthwhile endeavour.'*
> Pilates (1945, p11)

You can find Beginners' Pilates sessions by visiting YouTube.com and searching for my channel, 'Gila Archer Pilates'.

Pilates for posture

Rebalancing our posture is vital today as we spend more and more time bent forward over desks, computers and phones. It is this forward head posture and slumping over which places unnecessary tension and stress on neck and back muscles and reduces the space for our internal organs to function efficiently.

Even if you have an active job or play lots of sports most of us are not symmetrical. We have a strong side and a weak side, and Pilates exercises rebalance any of these discrepancies in our everyday movement which can lead to bad habits, our bodies not functioning as well as they could and aches and pains.

Get Moving

Stand up. Feet hip width apart, with your weight equally spread through your feet. Bring your pelvis into a neutral position (midway point).

Roll your shoulders up and then down, sliding your shoulder blades down into your back pockets. Bring your chin in slightly, lengthening the back of your neck and bringing your eyes, shoulders, hips, knees and ankle into a straight line.

Close your eyes if you want to and just take a moment to focus on how this posture feels.

Revisit it first thing in the morning, last thing at night and every now and then during the day.

Imagine I'm on your shoulder, reminding you about your posture!

Feel better?

You can find Posture Pilates sessions by visiting YouTube.com and searching for my channel, 'Gila Archer Pilates'.

Pilates for balance

Our ability to balance decreases as we age, and this can lead to us to being more likely to fall and injure ourselves. Our balance relies on our vision, our vestibular system (the system in our inner ear that provides feedback about our balance and spatial orientation) and our muscular system all working efficiently together. As our sight decreases, we must rely more on having the strength and awareness in our body to be able to avoid hazards, catch ourselves if we trip and respond quickly to right ourselves.

Practising our balance is a vital skill to maintain as we age. It is easy to bring balance into everything you do. You could do the washing up on one leg, brush your teeth on one leg or stand up to get dressed and put your trousers on.

Get Moving

Stand up. You are balancing! Now, have a go at closing your eyes. If you prefer, have a wall or something or someone you can hold onto nearby.

Notice how, without your vision, your proprioception (awareness of where your body is in space) is working harder. You may feel the muscles in your legs working, you may be swaying slightly. All of these are good signs – because your body is constantly using this awareness to keep you standing and not falling over.

Now, open your eyes, stand on one leg, arms crossed, and when you are ready, close your eyes again. Continue to have something or someone close by for support if you want to.

Notice how your supporting leg is making minute adjustments all the time to keep you standing. Now, try on the other leg. Does your other leg feel stronger or more wobbly?

You can find Balance Pilates sessions by visiting YouTube.com and searching for my channel, 'Gila Archer Pilates'.

Pilates for energy

Being part of a sedentary society, we can often feel lethargic. Many women have said to me that they just don't have enough energy to exercise – but this is backwards thinking, because when we move, we become more energised.

Focusing on our breathing during Pilates also has the advantage of bringing fresh air into the body and expelling stale air. The oxygen-rich fresh blood is then circulated to our muscles, organs and brain, helping to reenergise us.

> *"The exercises have stirred your sluggish circulation into action and to performing its duty more effectively in the matter of discharging fatigue-products created by your muscular and mental activities. Your brain clears and your will power function.'*
>
> Pilates (1945, p12)

Get Moving

Stand up. Take a deep breath in and sweep your arms up above your head, breathe out as you sweep your arms down. Repeat three times.

Take your legs slightly wider than hip width apart, gently sweep your arms across your body as you twist round to the right and then the left. You are creating a fluid spine twist. Look to the back of the room and exhale as you twist round.

Do this a few times, keeping arms low, then repeat with arms at shoulder height, then a few times with arms at a diagonal, pointing to the top of wall where it meets the ceiling. Bring your arms back to shoulder height, then low down, all the time twisting.

Feel better?

You can find Energising Pilates sessions by visiting YouTube.com and searching for my channel, 'Gila Archer Pilates'.

Pilates for strength

Our movement relies on strength, requiring our muscles to be strong enough to move the bones at their joints and our mind being strong enough to not give up and give in.

As we grow older, we can easily lose strength because we lose muscle mass. This is called sarcopenia. Less strength makes moving harder – even all those everyday tasks that when we are young we take for granted.

For many of us reading this book, we have designed ourselves a comfortable life. We have sofas, chairs with backs, cars and many labour-saving devices in all areas of our lives e.g., washing machines, tumble driers, shopping trolleys, suitcases with wheels and of course mobile phones and the internet. You don't even have to leave your house for food anymore – you can order it all from the comfort of your own home! Even more vital then, that we find ways to keep building our strength.

Pilates uses your own body weight as resistance, so you can build strength in a functional way. You don't need to use any weights or equipment. All you need is a mat.

> *'Pilates [Contrology] is not a system of haphazard exercises designed to produce only bulging muscles. There is a reason.'*
>
> Pilates (1945, p14)

Get Moving

Do The Hundred

This is a classic Pilates move which I've modified here so you can start to build your core strength.

1. Lay on your back with knees bent and feet flat on the floor, hip width apart.

2. Rock your pelvis forwards and backwards and find your midway point, your neutral spine.

3. Lift both knees into your chest and then make sure they are in line over your hips and that your shins are parallel to the floor, as if you were resting your legs on a coffee table.

4. Maintain your neutral spine. The weight of your legs will want to tilt the pelvis and hollow your spine and this is where the strength in your deep abdominals comes in – to maintain neutral.

5. Hold for 10 deep breaths.

Easier option:
~ Just lift one leg and hold for 5 breaths, then swap legs.

Harder options:
~ Lift your head, shoulders and arms off the floor, reaching fingertips down the side of your legs and looking through your knees.

~ Straighten legs.

You can find Strength Pilates sessions by visiting YouTube.com and searching for my channel, 'Gila Archer Pilates'.

Pilates for flexibility

As I've already mentioned earlier in this book, you need a balance of strength and flexibility. One without the other does not give you effective, functional movement.

You want to be able to tie your shoelaces, put on your socks, reach for your seatbelt in the car, turn to look to see if traffic is coming when you are driving, put your arm in the sleeve of your coat, do your bra up at your back – these all require flexibility in your muscles and mobility in your joints.

Pilates focuses on moving your body in all three planes of movement, and stretches your body where it is tight.

'Bulging muscles hinder the attainment of flexibility because the over-developed muscles interfere with the proper development of underdeveloped muscles. True flexibility can be achieved when all muscles are uniformly developed.'

Pilates (1945, p16)

Get Moving

Get some stripey socks, leggings or tights and put them on!

This is just a fun way of measuring your flexibility – but you can use your own method if you don't own any stripey clothing!

Sit, with your legs out straight in front of you and together. Reach forward gently and see how far you can reach – which colour stripe have you got to?

Then, keeping that stretch, flex your feet and you may notice the stretch increase. Hold for a moment, then point your feet and you'll feel the stretch ease. Reach a little bit further forward.

Repeat the flex, hold, point, hold 3 times.

Last time – have you managed to stretch to the next stripe?

You can find Pilates Stretch sessions by visiting YouTube.com and searching for my channel, 'Gila Archer Pilates'.

Pilates for back care

Humans have evolved to stand upright, and our spine therefore easily becomes compressed. The spine is a very complex structure with 33 individual bones that can all flex, extend, side bend, and rotate. Lack of movement in all three planes of movement through every part of the spine causes areas of our back to become stiff and stuck.

Osteopathic or chiropractic care is highly beneficial from the right practitioner to help release some of the fixations. But this is not enough on its own. Your spine needs to be moved actively as well as passively, meaning that while someone else can help get movement through your spine, you need to put movement through your spine as well in order to retrain your body.

Over my many years of teaching I have had countless people with backache who have been referred to me by osteopaths, chiropractors and doctors, and I support a number of my husband's patients on their road to recovery. Pilates improves the mobility in the joints of the spine and strengthens all the small, deep muscles around the spine to make it stronger too. Pilates movements are gentle and specific.

Pilates helped me recover from backache after I stopped training as a gymnast, during and after each pregnancy and when I was breastfeeding. A number of my clients have also found Pilates beneficial for relieving their backache, and continue to remain consistent with practising Pilates as they know prevention is better than cure. It's easier, less inconvenient and cheaper than surgery!

One of the best prescriptions for your back is movement.

Get Moving

Lay on your back, feet flat and knees bent.

Breathe in.

As you exhale, tuck your tail bone under, imprinting your spine on the floor and gradually peel your spine off, vertebra by vertebra, until your knees, hips and shoulder are in a gentle sloping line.

Breathe in at the top and then exhale as you walk your spine back down, piece by piece, in order, as if each vertebra were a pearl on a string of pearls.

Repeat three times.

If you suffer from backache or you know anyone who does, try out these back care Pilates sessions:

You can find Back Care Pilates sessions by visiting YouTube.com and searching for my channel, 'Gila Archer Pilates'.

Pilates for sleep

Many of us don't get enough sleep or sufficient good quality sleep in our modern world, often because our minds can be so busy and constantly stimulated that it's not easy to switch off.

We ignore our circadian rhythms and natural sleep patterns to fit in with the hours we work, when children go to school and other time constraints that are established in society.

Sleep is so, so important and I'd recommend Mathew Walker's book *Why We Sleep* if you are interested in learning more about this topic.

Pilates helps with our sleep in that it helps us to switch off from the busyness of the day, slowing our breathing and its gentle movements can be very relaxing and therapeutic.

I have many clients who always have a better night's sleep on the days that they have done Pilates.

One client loves this following Pilates sessions so much that she says she now does it before bed every evening because she just gets the best night's sleep and wakes feeling so rested.

I'd love you to try it:

You can find Pilates for Better Sleep sessions by visiting YouTube.com and searching for my channel, 'Gila Archer Pilates'.

Pilates as a break from your desk

If you have found your neck and back aching from sitting at your desk in one position for too long, again, Pilates is a great way to take a quick break from your desk and reset your posture.

'It was (Pilates) conceived and tested with the idea of properly and scientifically exercising every muscle in your body in order to improve the circulation of the blood so that the bloodstream can and will carry more and better blood to feed every fibre and tissue of your body.'

Pilates(1945, p14)

Get Moving

Give your eyes a break from reading this book. Stand up, find your nearest stairs and walk or run up and down them three times.

Stand on the bottom step, holding onto the wall and banister, toes on the step and heels off and as you bend one knee, then allow the other heel to drop down, thereby stretching out the calf.

Do this three times on each leg, keeping the leg straight, and then three times bending both legs and feel the stretch in a different place in the calf.

You can find 'Take a break from your desk' Pilates sessions by visiting YouTube.com and searching for my channel, 'Gila Archer Pilates'.

Pilates for pelvic floor

Our pelvic floor is often a subject that can be embarrassing to talk about, but whether we've had children or not, keeping our pelvic floor muscles working effectively is something we would all want. Our pelvic floor muscles need to be functional, both strong and able to relax.

Our pelvic floor is working all the time because of its relationship with our breathing. So, by focusing on our breathing, as we do in Pilates, we are also working the pelvic floor muscles. Our pelvic floor muscles are also part of what we call our 'Core' which is a fundamental part of everything we do in Pilates. By connecting with our core muscles, we are by default also connecting with our pelvic floor. Having said that, we can also have a focus on the pelvic floor muscles in a Pilates workout too.

Even as you are reading this book you can pause and focus your attention onto your pelvic floor for one minute.

Get Moving

Do 5 slow, long squeezes with your pelvic floor.

Do 5 short, quick squeezes.

Hold the pelvic floor contracted for a count of 10.

Pilates for pregnancy

Pilates is safe for most women during pregnancy and can help them keep fit, keep moving and take some time for self-care both during their pregnancy and post-partum. Moves are easily adapted to different positions and with the use of equipment as support if required.

Pilates can help with diastasis recti (separation of the two abdominal muscles or 6-pack muscles that run down the middle of the front of your body) that may occur during pregnancy, and help to reduce any gap between the abdominals and improve core strength.

I am intentionally not providing a general session here for any women that are pregnant or have just given birth because every woman's medical needs should be taken into consideration when planning them a Pilates session.

If you are interested in my support pre- or post-natal, please get in touch with me.

Pilates for arthritis

Pilates is a great choice if you suffer from arthritis. It is low impact and mobilises joints. Keeping moving helps to lubricate joints, relieve pain and maintain a range of movement. Pilates can also be specifically tailored to your individual needs.

You can find Gentle Mobility Pilates sessions by visiting YouTube.com and searching for my channel, 'Gila Archer Pilates'.

Pilates for when you're stuck, sat in the car waiting outside your children's activities

A number of my clients have said they are often sat for at least 30 minutes if not an hour or more in a car waiting outside their children's sports lessons and it's not always decent weather or an appropriate place to get out of your car and go for a walk. One client challenged me to see if I could put together a Pilates workout that you could do in the car!

So I did! It's a bitesize Pilates session you can do in your car, whatever the weather, so that you can make the most of your time and stop your back from aching or aimlessly scrolling through social media achieving nothing!

You can find my 'Pilates in the Car' session by visiting YouTube.com and searching for my channel, 'Gila Archer Pilates'.

Pilates if you just have absolutely no time whatsoever!

Well, as we've discussed earlier in this book, we now know we all have enough time, it's down to how we use it.

But I also know how life can be sometimes, so I have created a '1-Minute Pilates series' – and you can't tell me you can't find 1 minute, I just won't believe you.

Try out my '1-Minute Pilates' series.

You can find my '1-Minute Pilates' sessions by visiting YouTube.com and searching for my channel, 'Gila Archer Pilates'.

Pilates for life

Here are some fun challenges to help you to incorporate movement into your everyday life:

1. Stand on one leg whilst brushing your teeth: 1 minute right leg, 1 minute left leg.
2. Rise up on your toes and lower whilst washing up.
3. Make putting your arms in your coat sleeves into a spine twist, right and left.
4. Roll down through your spine whilst in the shower.
5. Do wall press-ups whilst waiting for kettle to boil.
6. Place your hands on the work surface in your kitchen, step back and allow your chest to open to the floor and then round the spine. Do this 3 or 4 times whilst cooking or waiting for the washing machine to spin out.
7. Stand up from the floor and sit back down on the floor without using your hands, knees or arms.
8. Play the game *Twister* with friends and family.
9. Engage your core and pelvic floor whilst sat at your desk, waiting at a red traffic light or pushing a shopping trolley.
10. Squat down to pick things up from the floor and pick up one thing at a time!

Enjoy these and let me know how you get on!

You can find more ideas to incorporate Pilates into your everyday life by visiting my website and downloading your own copy of my free booklet: *33 Quick and Easy Ways to Incorporate Pilates into your Everyday Life*.

There are many more topics and areas of the body I could cover, but I've selected the ones which I feel may be most relevant to those of you reading this book.

If there is something I haven't mentioned that you would like me to cover, I am always open to suggestions, so please get in touch and I'll see what I can do to support you.

You can of course check out my YouTube channel to find more workouts, along with all the ones I've already referred to. Go to YouTube and type in 'Gila Archer Pilates' and you'll find me there.

Get Thinking

The range of workouts I've included are not designed to overwhelm you, but to help address some specific needs that Pilates can help with and which in my experience are quite common.

Which workout are you going to do first?

Leave me a message/comment when you've done it so I can hear how you've got on.

Please note: You don't need a YouTube account to access any of the videos.

Chapter 7

You're a super woman – not Superwoman

Did you ever want to be Wonder Woman when you were younger?

Ever wish you had magic powers?

This scenario is something my children and I often discuss: if you could choose a magic power, what would it be?

I'd love to be as flexible as Elastigirl from *The Incredibles*. I'd love to be able to turn invisible, just to hide from my children and win hide and seek! I'd also like to be able to multiply and clone more of me, like the baby in *The Incredibles*, so I could actually do 5 things at once!

Wouldn't it be great to have super powers?

Wonder Woman is gifted with her powers from the gods. She gained beauty from Aphrodite, strength from Demeter, wisdom from Athena, speed and flight from Hermes, advanced senses and unity with beasts from Artemis and the ability to discern the truth from Hestia.

Her top powers are:

1. Immortality: she does not age beyond her prime.
2. Advanced sense: she can detect her enemies from a distance, is able to deflect bullets and fight even with a blindfold on.
3. Supreme strength: she can bend objects, break through buildings and lift vehicles.
4. Supreme stamina: she never tires.
5. Mind control: she is capable of commanding whole armies using just the power of her mind, and when she has a god or mortal wrapped in the lasso of Hestia, they are bound to tell the absolute truth.
6. Healing power: she can heal minor and major wounds within seconds.
7. Flight and speed: she can think, react, move and run at superhuman speed, she can defy gravity and leap and fly in the air.
8. Animal empathy: she can communicate and calm all forms of animals when needed.

Just take a look at all those powers. I'd like to put it to you that we, as women, have our own set of powers and some are not dissimilar to those of Wonder Woman. It might just be that some we are a bit out of practice in using.

1. ***Healing powers:*** As a mother and a woman we help to heal other people's wounds whether physical or mental. As a child, if I'd hurt myself the only person who could 'make it better' was my mum. As an adult, when I had to have surgery from an ectopic pregnancy, the only person I wanted to see was my mum. As a mother myself now, I have cared for and nurtured my children through every fall, stumble and worry.

   As a teacher, I have helped children up when they have fallen over, I've helped them to have courage to learn and try new things and I've listened when they've been upset.

   As a sister, I have listened and helped my sister in times of need.

As a daughter I have been there for my parents when their parents passed away.

As a granddaughter, I have listened and talked to my Nanna so she has had some company.

As a wife, I have listened and supported my husband through times of need.

So, as a woman, you have healing powers, and you use them all the time without probably even realising it.

2. ***Advanced senses:*** As women we have evolved to be aware of everything around us. Whereas male ancestors had to be able to focus and block out distractions to be effective in a hunt, our female ancestors had to be constantly looking around us as we foraged for berries, plants, water and of course keep an eye on the young. We are tuned in to being aware of other people's body language, their feelings and the things that are unsaid.

I'm sure you've heard the saying that women have eyes in the back of their head – well it's true!

Have you ever sensed that someone is unhappy or needs help without them saying?

Do you wake up the split second before your baby starts crying?

Do you detect when your 7-year-old is trying to tiptoe down the stairs because he should really be in bed?

Do you know when your children or an adult is lying to you?

Do you notice the toddler in a busy room about to grab the hot drink that's been left almost in reach when no-one else does?

These are your advanced senses.

3. **Strength:** We all have a strength within us and I'm sure you've heard of stories where 'ordinary' women have lifted cars in order to save their child. In 2012, Laura Kornacki, a 22-year-old, raised a BMW off her father when the car toppled from a jack.

Have you ever felt that 'fire' in you when your children, parents or loved ones are threatened in some way? Your instinct kicks in to protect and save them.

We are strong physically and mentally – all the strength we need is within us.

4. **Stamina:** I'm not thinking stamina to run miles or fight off enemies, but stamina to keep going. Even when you're tired from many sleepless nights you still get up to feed or change your baby or sit up all night with your poorly child or poorly pet. Even when YOU are feeling poorly you carry on.

5. **Mind control:** As you now know, your mind is truly powerful, you are the creator of your thoughts, and you can choose which thoughts to focus on.

As a teacher I became very good at the 'teacher look'. My mum was a teacher and was a master at this look and if she used the 'teacher look' on us as children we knew not to push things any further. My little brother would always dramatically collapse on the floor whenever my mum did the 'teacher look'!

I became quite skilled with this look too and could silence a whole class by just looking at them this way. If you are a teacher, I'm sure you'll know exactly what I mean, or you may have experienced this look from a teacher or your mum when you were younger.

My daughter, who is only 9, has the ability to produce this powerful look too!

With your mind you can change your world and how you see it. It may take some practice if you are out of the habit of using your powers – but they are there. As we explored in Chapter 4, with the right mindset you can achieve anything you want to.

*6. **Immortality:*** Well, some people say age is just a number, as you are as old as you feel. So, as long as in our minds we feel in our prime, then we are and we live on in our legacies that we leave behind, whether that be in our children, our families, our friends, our work, our purpose, and all those who we have helped in our time here.

*7. **Flight and speed:*** OK, I will admit that we may not be able to fly like a bird, but let's think outside the box. We all can fly. Fly out of our comfort zones and into the world that holds our potential, one that is full of magic and possibilities. I was bought a fridge magnet as a present once by one of my pupils. I still have it. It says, 'All children are born with wings. Teachers help them to fly'. This is true for all of us. We all have wings and can learn to fly with the help of others and by taking that first step out of the nest. As for speed, we can all move forward and it doesn't matter at what speed that is, because progress is progress. You know the story of the tortoise and the hare, right? It's about maintaining a consistent speed and continuing to take the right next step.

So often, we put pressure on ourselves to be Superwoman. To do everything, perfectly, be in two places at once and never need to rest. As we have just explored, there are many powers that as women we possess. But like any superhero, you are not perfect. And you don't need to be. You are human, a woman, and with the powers you have, that is enough.

You are enough.

You are already a super, awesome woman, with your own powers and qualities that can be added to the ones above that make you, you.

You can add 'Do Pilates' because that is a super power too! I have a t-shirt that says, 'I do Pilates. What's your super power?' So, it must be true!

Get Thinking

What are your top 10 powers? List them below

1.
2.
3.
4.
5.
6.
7.
8.
9.
10.

When I tried to be Superwoman and meet society's and some other people's expectations, I was left drained physically and mentally and I was unkind to myself.

I felt I had to be able to do everything. I would make World Book Day character costumes instead of buying them, telling myself that buying them was too easy an option. I did absolutely everything for my wedding, from making invitations and my cake to decorating the venue, organising gifts, guests, place settings, dresses and suits, flowers etc. I never liked my children missing their activities, so if something clashed one week, I would desperately rush around aiming to be in two places at once. I would plan the meals for the week, go to the supermarket, cook the dinner and make puddings. I would do washing, tidying and cleaning, gardening, rubbish bins, and so on. I never took the time to even think about what to wear; I'd just throw on the same clothes that I'd worn the day before, as if I didn't matter. You get the idea.

I never once asked for help. I believed asking for help was a sign of me failing. I didn't want to fail – that wasn't an option.

But the outcome was that I was not Superwoman but a frazzled, tired, overwhelmed, grumpy, irritable, unhappy woman who wasn't using her powers at all, but allowing life to take over control.

I am so glad I have now taken back hold of the reins and am using my powers again. My mind control is stronger, and every day I am becoming a better version of myself. I am a super, awesome woman in my own right. I am being the person I want to be and getting better every day.

You have nothing to prove to society, to your parents, your family, your friends or your colleagues.

Be your best self for you because you are important too.

You are a super woman.

At the start of this book, I explained how I felt lost for a time, and I've been on a journey ever since to find my best self.

Here is a visual representation of the journey I and many other women are on and each of our journeys look slightly different, and we are all at different points on that journey. You may be just at the start or have taken a few steps forward only to feel like you've come to a standstill or you're not sure how to continue further.

Your Best Self Pathway

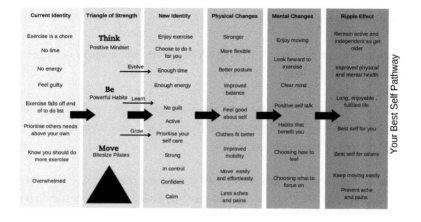

Get Moving

Do something active today that you **enjoy** doing, e.g., Pilates, walking, swimming, gardening, running, climbing, playing sport, dancing, cycling, skipping, jumping on a trampoline. Anything that involves moving your body and you enjoy doing. Do it for you!

I've shared with you my transformation in my many stories in this book and so I'd now like to share with you some Pilates journey stories from some of my clients.

Sarah's Pilates journey

Sarah was a conscientious hard worker. She had two children and was the main breadwinner in her family. Over the years she had done some swimming and some running, but she would only stick with these for a few months at a time.

She worked from home and after her husband left to take the children to school, she'd switch on her computer and start working. It would be about 8.30am even though she didn't officially have to start work until 9.00am.

She would often eat her lunch at her desk and not take a break until the children arrived home or she took them to their after-school clubs. By the time she got back in she felt too tired and unmotivated to do any exercise, preferring to collapse on the sofa with a glass of wine.

When her back started aching and twingeing and she was living with increasing pain, she decided enough was enough and sought out my help.

Since working with me, she has recognised that she was working longer hours without the need, recognition or reward for doing so, and not allowing herself time to exercise. She changed her routine and started work at 9.00am which was when she was supposed to start work and used the time from when the children left for school until she started work to do a bitesize Pilates session and make herself a nutritious breakfast.

As a result, she spent the rest of the day feeling very pleased with herself, that she had achieved this. She'd done her exercise for the day and wasn't left having endless discussions with herself about whether she should do it or not. Her confidence in her own abilities grew and in how she moved. She could pick up the washing basket without worrying about her back going. She could sit at her desk for longer more comfortably. She has taken responsibility for herself and for her health and fitness.

Joan's Pilates journey

Joan is in her 70s and joined my weekly Pilates classes over 14 years ago because she'd had knee surgery and wanted to rebuild the strength in her leg. Although the doctor had said she would need surgery on the other knee the following year, she was keen to avoid that if she could. During the classes, I'd always adapt any kneeling exercises as it was uncomfortable for her to put weight on her knee, and she had limited range of movement in the knee joint.

She had always been active, enjoying swimming and walking but knew as she got older, she wanted to be able to continue enjoying these activities and the social aspects as well. As a widower, it was important for her to continue to go out and remain active and independent.

Joan is now a member of CORE and says she has never felt stronger. She never needed her second knee surgery and I no longer adapt any kneeling exercises. She can confidently work in a kneeling position and even sit back on her heels with a good range of movement in both knees. She continues to walk and swim, look after grandchildren and dogs, and truly is an inspiration to remaining committed and consistent.

Hannah's Pilates journey

Hannah has three children and runs her own business. She was always very busy and felt doing any exercise for herself was selfish.

It wasn't until she started following me that she realised how she'd been getting in her own way and putting obstacles up to doing any exercise because she believed she had to look after everyone else first.

If I remember correctly, it was when I gave her the analogy of being in a plane and the oxygen masks drop, that you put on your own oxygen mask first before you help others otherwise you are not capable of helping anyone else, that she started to shift her perspective.

I remember her saying to me that she now gives herself permission to do her bitesize Pilates. She knows that if she misses a workout on one day, that's OK, she can pick up again the next day. There is no guilt or giving herself a hard time. Because she is now being consistent with her exercise and being kind to herself with her thoughts, her flexibility has increased, and her upper body strength has improved.

Susan's Pilates journey

Susan is a mum of a toddler and runs her own business. She is very proud of the fact that she is organised, well planned, makes decisions, employs people, manages a team and juggles lots of balls to help her clients.

However, several years ago, her back started hurting and it was stopping her being able to concentrate at work and sit for long periods of time. She wished she could lift her child up without her back going and she wanted to be able to have a restful night's sleep without her back aching.

After visiting doctors and physiotherapists she was recommended to do Pilates and she found me.

I've helped her over the last few years to stop putting her exercise off in favour of work. She understands why she wants to exercise and is motivated to not just relieve the pain but in preventing going back to how she was living. She has become a role model for her child and now easily fits her bitesize Pilates into her schedule.

When she has fallen off track, she has sought my help and with my support has picked it back up, knowing that her progress won't be smooth, there will be days when her back may still ache, but she is learning to be patient and persistent. She now has an established routine and is feeling the benefits of doing Pilates regularly.

Dorothy's Pilates journey

Dorothy had struggled for over 10 years with back pain that meant she had to give up work and could not sit down. She had visited osteopaths, physiotherapists and doctors, and she had gained some movement in her back but was still not able to work.

I worked with her for many months, helping her to improve her movement. The biggest change came when I asked her to focus on what she could do and had improved on. For so many years she had focused on the restriction in her back, on the pain it caused and how it stopped her doing things that she had become very hard on herself and kept her attention on what she wasn't able to do.

With my support she shifted her perspective and focused on what she *was* able to do. She became more positive and confident in how she moved. She could bend down to pick something off the floor with ease and fluidity. She was able to sit for almost an hour and was considering a phased return to work. Her mindset, along with regular, consistent, specific movement through the Pilates I taught her, has given her the beginnings of what will become a huge ripple effect. She is at the start of her Pilates journey, and her momentum will build. I'm really excited for what she will experience in the next few years.

None of these women that I've talked about are Superwoman – but they are super women. They are the same as you and me. We are all at different stages in our journey and we are all moving forward together.

Get Thinking

Imagine your best self...

Close your eyes and picture yourself, what you are doing, how you are being, what you are wearing, what you look like, what your life looks like – what powers do you have?

Now write these down or draw them. Describe the person you want to be, and that may include using some of those powers you have but have forgotten about.

What will your ripple effect be? In one year's time what will your life look like? Imagine a secret camera in your house, what would I see and hear? How would your life look?

Describe or draw it.

What about in 5 years' time?

Being a woman is in itself a superpower. Step into your power.

Chapter 8

There's more to life than Pilates

*H*ow I met Joe!

Joseph Pilates and I met many years ago. I had started doing his exercises before I even knew it was him behind them. I bought his book, *Return to Life through Contrology* which he signed for me!

After retiring from gymnastics, Pilates was there for me and has been with me every step of my journey since. Joe continues to inspire me and long may my love affair with Pilates continue. Even when I did no exercise for myself, when I struggled to enjoy moving, Pilates was still a part of my life. By continuing to teach Pilates throughout each of my three pregnancies I kept moving and I kept helping other women to move better.

I love being able to move. I love feeling strong, flexible and confident. I love being able to still challenge my mind and my body by doing physical activities that I enjoy: ballet and aerial silks. I love being upside down – you get a different perspective on the world when you are upside down!

None of that would be possible without Joe by my side!

There is more to life than Pilates though. And I think Joseph would agree. Pilates unlocks your potential to move better and thus enjoy leading a fulfilling and physically active life.

And that is why I am still in love with Pilates over 20 years on.

My journey continues and so does yours. Enjoy your journey and have fun in moving.

Get Moving

Choose to do something active today that you enjoy. It can be something you already do, or how about finding something new, that you've always wanted to be better at or learn? Have a go, for example, maybe at ice-skating, pole dancing, gravy wrestling (yes, that is a thing – one of my Pilates clients entered herself into the annual championships a few years ago), boxing, cricket, badminton – whatever you enjoy!

My journey started with movement as a huge part of my life, so much so that I won gold medals, performed at national levels, on stage, achieved high grades and felt invincible. My lifestyle changed when I had three children under the age of 4 and I devoted my time to them. As a result, I neglected myself, was unkind to myself and beat myself up because I had stopped moving. My journey was not plain sailing, I had ups and downs and every time I had good intentions to start moving again, I would, without realising, sabotage my good intentions.

I am, however, very grateful for everything I have learnt about myself through this journey and that I can now share with you, so you can enjoy your journey of moving better and feeling alive again. It won't take you as long as it took me, because I was finding the path which I can now guide you along.

11 years after my first child was born, I now feel so much better about myself. I have regained my confidence in moving, regained my core strength after having three children, maintained my flexibility and choose to do Pilates because I enjoy it. It doesn't take over my life but enables me to continue living my life to the full. I am a confident, calm and professional woman who has the energy, physical capability and mental clarity to decide to live my life on purpose, and that life is active, healthy and fulfilled.

I have changed in how I show up, how I walk, what I say to myself and when I am asked, "Hi Gila, how are you?" I reply, "I'm feeling really great thank you. How are you?"

When asked to introduce myself or tell people a bit more about me, it is now comfortable and automatic for me to say, "Hi, I'm Gila and I'm an entrepreneur. I help busy women, whose fitness feels like another chore on their never-ending to-do list, to live an active and fulfilled life by teaching them my unique approach: 'B.E.S.T. – Best Empowered Self Triangle'. I am a Level 4 Pilates Instructor, Primary School Teacher, Movement Expert, wife, mum of three children, ballet dancer, aerial silks artist, lover of all things chocolate and now – a published author!"

What a difference to the woman who a few years ago described herself as a busy mum who helped her husband with his business.

It's that unique combination of how I think – having a positive mindset, how I am being; having powerful habits and how I am moving – and having bitesize Pilates as the foundation of my movement routine, that has empowered and enabled me to become the best version of myself.

I want this for you too.

Get Thinking

What would you like to be able to do with the remainder of your life?

What movement goals do you have? Don't overthink them, just write them down.

List and brainstorm everything you'd really like to do, learn or try. This could be a new sport, a physical experience, enjoying living your life and doing what you currently do but more easily and maybe for longer e.g., walking/gardening. It may be that your goal is that you want to feel good about yourself, or that you'd like to enjoy moving.

What do you need to change or do differently to achieve these goals?

Now, I want to be transparent with you though and not give you any false impression that this has been an easy, straightforward journey, nor one that I knew where it would lead me. It would be easy to look at fitness influencers on social media and assume that they have achieved everything they have by themselves. You know that I am not Superwoman and therefore could not have achieved this without help and support from a lot of people over several years. I've made mistakes but those mistakes have enabled me to grow.

I have not travelled my journey alone. So many people have touched my life and helped me get to where I am now, some of whom I've never met! These are the main people who have helped me: my husband, children, parents, siblings, colleagues in the fitness industry, entrepreneurs in business and coaching, my VA, my ballet teacher, my silks instructor, my gymnastic coach, my colleagues in education, my writing coach, Joseph Pilates (and all chocolate manufacturers – the consumption of a fair amount of chocolate along the way has helped me too!!!!!!)

In my first job as a teacher, I was one of a team of 5 awesome women. Each with our own unique skills, talents and powers. We were all brilliant on our own, but as a team we were even stronger. There was no element of competition between us. We were all working towards the same goal – which was to teach the children in that year group to the best of our abilities and champion each other's strengths.

You knew they would have your back if something went wrong. You knew if you were having a bad day, they would be there to listen. You knew they would support you, encourage you to develop and share your strengths. Looking back, I am so grateful I got to experience working in such a team and fulfilling my potential as a teacher and as a woman. Thank you to these ladies for the best 7 years of my teaching career, and they will know who they are if they read this.

Women are powerful individuals, but together we have impact.

Get Thinking

Write down something big that you have achieved in your life.

Did you do it on your own or with help? Who helped you?

Chances are you had help and support. Am I right?

You don't have to do it alone

1 **Have a team around you.** Surround yourself with like-minded women who genuinely want you to do well. It will make a huge difference to your success and progress.

'Surround yourself with people who have habits you want to have yourself. You'll rise together.' Clear (2018, p117)

2. **Be brave and ask for help.** Asking for help is not a sign of failing or not being good enough. It's a sign of knowing yourself, what your strengths are and having the courage and confidence to ask for help. We all have our own powers, our own unique qualities, so let's use each other's strengths and be stronger together.

3. **Remember, it's not about staying on your horse.** Everyone falls off at times, but it's about how quickly you can get back on. The only people who fail are the ones that give up.

4. **Have an accountability partner.** Work with someone who is an expert in their field, who has your back (quite literally in the case of Pilates!) and wants this for you as much as you do.

5. **Believe in yourself.** Tell yourself you can do it, because I know you can.

It is within yourself that you have the strength you need.

Celebrate!

So, let me finish here by first of all saying congratulations for reading this book and completing the **Get Thinking** and **Get Moving** action steps along the way.

Just by doing this you have already made huge progress and will have shifted your perspective about yourself, your mind and your body. You have begun your Pilates lifestyle. Acknowledge that commitment you made to yourself at the start of this book, acknowledge what you have achieved so far and take a moment to celebrate it!

How do you like to celebrate?

(Me, I sometimes like to celebrate with my favourite chocolate or a good book in a hot bubble bath with the door locked! And other times I like to celebrate with my family.)

What now?

You are almost at the end of this book, so what happens now? Do you say, great book Gila, put it on the bookshelf, forget about it and go back to being a woman with no time or energy to take responsibility for her health and fitness?

Or

Are you going to continue on your journey with Pilates as part of your lifestyle, becoming the best version of yourself?

Get Thinking

What things have you already changed, become aware of, started doing differently as a result of reading this book? List them here.

Wow! Just take a moment to look back at this progress. You've done this pretty much on your own so far, so imagine how your life could look as you continue with support from me and other like-minded women.

If this book has helped you in any way, I would love to continue to help you along your journey and already feel privileged to be a part of it by you picking up my book and reading it. So, thank you.

Here is how I can continue to support you:

- Visit my YouTube channel, 'Gila Archer Pilates'. Please subscribe so I can continue to help you.
- Join my Facebook page 'Gila Archer Pilates' and Facebook Group: 'Bitesize Pilates for Busy Women'
- My website is full of advice and tips: www.gilaarcherpilates.com
- Join my Bitesize Pilates for Busy Women 6-week programme
- Subscribe to CORE – my online Pilates membership
- Find out about my 1-to-1 support, online or in person

My expertise is in movement and in helping women to move better. I am told that I am an awesome teacher, and I don't need to tell you that you are more likely to be successful if have the right support from the right people.

I'd love to hear how you've enjoyed this book and how it has helped change your life for the better.

Any questions, please just get in touch. My email address is gila@gilaarcherpilates.com

Don't underestimate the power of movement.

Enjoying and living a Pilates lifestyle can make you feel strong, healthy and fabulous!

Appendix

Some definitions

Here are some definitions I've found to describe movement:

Movement: The act or process of moving people or things from one place or position to another.

Exercise: Voluntary activity to sustain or improve our health and fitness, planned, structured and repetitive.

Physical activity: Any bodily movement produced by skeletal muscles that requires energy expenditure.

Sport: An activity involving physical exertion and skill in which an individual or team competes against another or others for entertainment.

Physical literacy: The motivation, confidence, physical competence, understanding and knowledge that individuals develop in order to maintain physical activity at an appropriate level throughout their life. Whitehead (2010)

Physical development: Growth and development of brain and body; developing control of muscles and physical co-ordination.

Principles of Pilates

Alignment: Correct alignment and posture are key to safe and effective practice.

Breathing: Correct breathing helps to provide a focus for your mind as it increases your oxygen intake. 'Breathing is the first act of life and the last. Our very life depends on it.' Pilates (1945, p13)

Centring: Stability in the centre enables grace and precision without any unwanted or unnecessary movement.

Concentration: The goal in Pilates is to focus on the present and be aware and mindful of the quality of all movement.

Co-ordination: Starting with simple movements and co-ordinating the breathing and then progressing movements by including adding in of the arms and legs.

Control: The mind and body work together to control movement.

Precision: Attention must be paid to detail. Think about the alignment of your body.

Flow: The effortless flow of movement seen in a skilled athlete or dancer.

Just by moving your body in a specific way, as done through Pilates exercises, you can build the strength you need to move easily and efficiently.

Acknowledgements

I'd like to thank everyone who has helped me on my journey so far and made this book become a reality.

Thank you

- ~ to Georgia, for seeing the best in me, even when I couldn't.
- ~ to Jo, who told me what I needed to hear.
- ~ to Sam, for making my book come to life.
- ~ to Mark, for editing and making sense of my book.
- ~ to my Pilates clients, for choosing me to help them enjoy moving and feel fabulous.
- ~ to Tulay, for her support and positive energy.
- ~ to J, for his unconditional love and support.
- ~ to T, D and B, for just being you and making my world complete.

Bibliography

Books

Blythe, Catherine (2018) *Enjoy Time*

Clear, James (2018) *Atomic Habits*

Connell, Gill and McCarthy, Cheryl (2014) *A Moving Child is a Learning Child: How the body teaches the brain to think*

Covey, Stephen (2004) *The 7 Habits of Highly Effective People*

Goddard Blythe, Sally (2009) *Attention Balance and Coordination – the A B C of Learning Success*

Goddard Blythe, Sally (2005) *The Well Balanced Child*

Goddard Blythe, Sally (2011) *The Genius of Natural Childhood*

Goddard Blythe, Sally (2008) *What Babies and Children Really Need*

Gallahue and Ozmun (1995) *Understanding Motor Development*

Hayden, Elizabeth C. (2000) 3rd ed *Osteopathy for Children*

Hornibrook, F. A (1929) *The Culture of the Abdomen*

Jeffers, Susan (2012) *Feel the Fear and Do It Anyway*

Jenkinson, Sally (2012) *The Genuis of Play*

Lieberman, Daniel (2021) *Exercised: the Science of Physical Activity, Rest and Health*

Matthews, Michael (2018) *The Little Black Book of Workout Motivation*

Nurse, Angela D (2009) *Physical Development in the Early Years Foundation Stage*

Piek, Jan (2006) *Infant Motor Development*

Pilates, Joseph (1945) *Return to Life through Contrology*

Pilates, Joseph (1934) *Your Health*

Sincero, Jen (2013) *You are a Badass*

Tracy, B (2017) *Eat That Frog*

Walker, Mathew (2018) *Why We Sleep*

Whitehead, M (2010) *Physical Literacy: Throughout the Lifecourse*

Websites

Gila Archer Pilates:
www.gilaarcherpilates.com

Alaska Sleep:
www.alaskasleep.com/blog/baby-sleep-position-affects-motor-development

British Heart Foundation:
www.bhf.org.uk/informationsupport/heart-matters-magazine/activity/sitting-down

British Medical Journal:
www.bmj.com/company/newsroom/spending-too-much-time-sitting-down-linked-to-around-50000-deaths-per-year-in-the-uk/

Dr Tulay Massey:
www.tulaymasseycoaching.com

Dyspraxia Foundation:
www.dyspraxiafoundation.org.uk/

Jo Davison:
www.jodavison.com

Just Stand:
www.juststand.org

NHS:
www.nhs.uk/conditions/baby/caring-for-a-newborn/reduce-the-risk-of-sudden-infant-death-syndrome/

NHS:
www.nhs.uk/live-well/exercise/

Safe to Sleep:

www.safetosleep.nichd.nih.gov/activities/campaign

Sleep Foundation:

www.sleepfoundation.org/insomnia/exercise-and-insomnia

Squatty Potty:

www.squattypotty.com

World Health Organisation:

www.who.int/health-topics/physical-activity#tab=tab_1

Pilates Foundation:

www.pilatesfoundation.com/pilates/the-history-of-pilates

Alma Osteopathic Practice YouTube Channel:

https://www.youtube.com/channel/UCzdBDvUtsttEKsQRlTC0H7Q

Journals / Articles

L C Argenta 1, L R David, J A Wilson, W O Bell (1996) *An increase in infant cranial deformity with supine sleeping position* https://pubmed.ncbi.nlm.nih.gov/9086895/

Sarah Louise Bell, Suzanne Audrey, David Gunnell, Ashley Cooper & Rona Campbell (2019) *The relationship between physical activity, mental wellbeing and symptoms of mental health disorder in adolescents: a cohort study* https://ijbnpa.biomedcentral.com/articles/10.1186/s12966-019-0901-7

Jen Campbell (2016) *Why Crawling is Important for your Baby* https://www.nationwidechildrens.org/family-resources-education/700childrens/2016/11/why-crawling-is-important-for-your-baby

Beth Ellen Davis, MD; Rachel Y. Moon, MD; Hari C. Sachs, MD; Mary C. Ottolini, MD (1998) Effects of Sleep Position on Infant Motor Development https://publications.aap.org/pediatrics/article-abstract/102/5/1135/61959/Effects-of-Sleep-Position-on-Infant-Motor

Claire Dewey, MSc; Peter Fleming, MB; Jean Golding, PhD; the ALSPAC Study Team (1998) *Does the Supine Sleeping Position Have Any Adverse Effects on the Child? II. Development in the First 18 Months* https://publications.aap.org/pediatrics/article-abstract/101/1/e5/52337/Does-the-Supine-Sleeping-Position-Have-Any-Adverse

Ben Godde and Claudia Voelcker-Rehage (2010) *More automation and less cognitive control of imagined walking movements in high versus low fit older adults.* https://www.ncbi.nlm.nih.gov/pmc/articles/PMC2944669/

Gries, K et al (2018) Cardiovascular and skeletal muscle health with lifelong exercise https://journals.physiology.org/doi/full/10.1152/japplphysiol.00174.2018

Harvard Health Publishing (2019) *The dangers of sitting* https://www.health.harvard.edu/pain/the-dangers-of-sitting

Kathy Katella (2019) *Why Is Sitting so Bad for Us?* https://www.yalemedicine.org/news/sitting-health-risks

Anthea Levi (2016) Why Crawling Is the Ultimate Total-Body Exercise https://www.health.com/fitness/crawling-core-exercise

Eric Martinsen (2009) *Physical Activity in the treatment of anxiety and depression* https://www.tandfonline.com/doi/full/10.1080/08039480802315640

New York Times: www.nytimes.com/2020/04/13/parenting/baby/tummy-time

Gary O'Donovan et al (2017) *Association of "Weekend Warrior" and Other Leisure Time Physical Activity Patterns With Risks for All-Cause, Cardiovascular Disease, and Cancer Mortality* https://jamanetwork.com/journals/jamainternalmedicine/fullarticle/2596007

John Persing, MD; Hector James, MD; Jack Swanson, MD; John Kattwinkel, MD; (2003) *Prevention and Management of Positional Skull Deformities in Infants* https://publications.aap.org/pediatrics/article-abstract/112/1/199/63410/Prevention-and-Management-of-Positional-Skull

W D Schmidt, C J Biwer, L K Kalscheuer (2001) *Effects of long versus short bout exercise on fitness and weight loss in overweight females.* https://pubmed.ncbi.nlm.nih.gov/11601564/

Dr. Jeremy Schmoe, DC DACNB FACFN FABBIR (2022) *Crawling is Important for Childhood Brain Development* https://thefnc.com/research/crawling-is-important-for-childhood-brain-development/

The Local (2016) *Norway school swaps chairs for rubber balls* https://www.thelocal.no/20160321/norway-school-swaps-chairs-for-giant-rubber-balls/

University of Birmingham (2018) *A lifetime of regular exercise slows down aging* https://www.sciencedaily.com/releases/2018/03/180308143123.htm

Tyler Wheeler (2022) *Why Sitting Too Much Is Bad for Your Health* https://www.webmd.com/fitness-exercise/ss/slideshow-sitting-health

Resources

33 quick and easy ways to incorporate Pilates into your everyday life (free ebook)
https://www.gilaarcherpilates.com/33-ways-to-integrate-pilates-movement-into-your-everyday-life

Gila Archer Pilates YouTube channel:
www.youtube.com search '*Gila Archer Pilates*'

Heartfelt Gratitude Audio from Tulay Massey Coaching
https://www.tulaymasseycoaching.com/heartfelt-gratitude-audio-Gila

Deformational Plagiocephaly & Cranial Remolding in Infants
https://pediatricapta.org/includes/fact-sheets/pdfs/Plagiocephaly.pdf

Top Tips for Tummy Time
https://www.nct.org.uk/baby-toddler/your-childs-development/0-3-months/top-tips-for-tummy-time

How to encourage your baby to crawl
https://www.sproutandthrive.com/blog/tag/crawling+linked+to+writing

Guide to Baby Wearing: Benefits, Safety Tips, and How To (2019)
https://www.healthline.com/health/parenting/baby-wearing#benefits

Sitting Calculator
https://www.juststand.org/the-tools/sitting-time-calculator/